The editors

Hans L. Rieder

Hans L. Rieder specialized in epidemiology and public health. After training in infectious diseases at Zurich University, he worked as a tuberculosis clinician in Thailand and then trained as a tuberculosis epidemiologist at the Centers for Disease Control and Prevention in the USA. He obtained his Master's degree in public health at Emory University, Atlanta, USA. He subsequently worked for the public health service in Switzerland before joining The Union, focusing on tuberculosis education and operations research. He is concurrently Senior Lecturer at the Universities of Berne and Zurich.

Chiang Chen-Yuan

Chiang Chen-Yuan is a qualified pulmonologist. After training in respiratory and critical care medicine at the National Taiwan University Hospital and Chronic Disease Control Bureau, Department of Health, he worked as a clinician, treating drug-resistant tuberculosis and lung diseases, and as departmental head of the national tuberculosis programme in Taiwan. Subsequently, he was trained by The Union (Donald Enarson) in international tuberculosis control and obtained a Master's degree in public health at the University of California, Berkeley, USA.

Robert P. Gie

Robert P. Gie trained in paediatrics with the Department of Paediatrics and Child Health, Stellenbosch University, South Africa. He currently works in the same department, where he heads the Paediatric Intensive Care and Paediatric Pulmonology units. He is attached to the Desmond Tutu Tuberculosis Centre, and has a major interest in the diagnosis and management of intrathoracic tuberculosis in children.

Donald A. Enarson

Donald A. Enarson is Senior Advisor to The Union in Paris. He qualified in medicine in Canada in 1970 and gained a specialist qualification in internal medicine in 1978. He worked in development programmes in Sudan and in the Philippines before entering academic medicine, becoming Professor of Medicine at the University of Alberta in 1987 and has held the post of Adjunct Professor there since 1993. His research has focused on tuberculosis and occupational lung diseases. He has been a public health advisor to the Ministries of Health, health services and development agencies for more than 40 countries.

Contents

Crofton's
Clinical Tuberculosis

Third Edition

Edited by:

Hans L. Rieder

International Union Against Tuberculosis and
Lung Disease, France

Chiang Chen-Yuan

International Union Against Tuberculosis and
Lung Disease, France

Robert P. Gie

Department of Paediatrics and Child Health,
Stellenbosch University, South Africa

Donald A. Enarson

International Union Against Tuberculosis and
Lung Disease, France

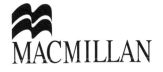

MACMILLAN

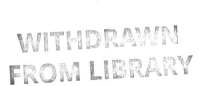

Macmillan Education
Between Towns Road, Oxford, OX4 3PP
A division of Macmillan Publishers Limited
Companies and representatives throughout the world

www.macmillan-africa.com

ISBN 978-1-4050-9737-6

First published 1993
Second edition 1998
This edition 2009

Design by Holbrook Design Oxford Ltd
Typeset by E Clicks Enterprise
Cover design by Charles Design Associates

Printed and bound in Malaysia

2013 2012 2011 2010 2009
10 9 8 7 6 5 4 3 2 1

Contents

Preface to the Third Edition

Much has changed since the first edition of this book was published in 1992. At that time, international efforts were focused on persuading decision makers and health service providers that, in spite of the general perception that tuberculosis was a 'passé' issue, it remained (and still remains) a substantial challenge globally and also locally, even in wealthy countries, where subsets of the population continue to experience risks of the disease in every way comparable to historical highs. The previous conception that 'tuberculosis is no longer a significant problem' has now hopefully been discredited and we will no longer see such statements in print.

Since the first edition was published, this text has been distributed widely throughout the world and has been received very positively by practitioners in every corner of the world. Wherever one goes, one finds 'Crofton's text' as a cornerstone for both practitioners and teachers. It has proved indispensable in bringing desperately needed assistance to those on the front lines of health services to provide the best possible care for their patients.

We have moved beyond the stage of having to persuade our colleagues and political leaders of the importance of tuberculosis, into a phase of rapid expansion of interest and engagement in the fight against this disease. This rapid expansion has seen immense resources mobilized and international agencies engaging in the global 'Stop TB Strategy'. The scope of the work has enlarged to address the huge challenges represented by the epidemic of the human immunodeficiency virus (HIV), the awareness of hard-to-manage multidrug-resistant tuberculosis and a wider awareness of the context of tuberculosis services, particularly the declining role of, and diminishing human resources in, the public sector, the woeful state of general health services, the deplorable poverty and social inequality where tuberculosis finds its home, and the promise (and delays) of 'new tools' with which to wage the fight against this historical foe.

This third edition reminds us that none of the wider issues matter unless we get the basics right. Preventing tuberculosis remains (in spite of all the promises of new strategies and tools) primarily a matter of providing high-quality care to individual patients. For this, 'Crofton's book' has been a guiding light and, hopefully, this third edition will carry on its glorious tradition. We provide this text in the sincere hope that it will arm hard-pressed service providers with the knowledge and skills necessary to carry on the most basic function of tuberculosis control – care of the patient.

Foreword to the Third Edition

Some years ago my two close friends and fellow authors, Fred Miller and Norman Horne, sadly passed away. I myself moved into my nineties. I therefore asked Professor Don Enarson if he would be prepared to update a third edition through the Union. He in turn asked Hans Rieder, who had given us much help with the second edition, to participate and to organize the work. They asked two other distinguished colleagues, Chiang Chen-Yuan and Robert Gie, to join them.

I have read their third edition with deep interest and admiration. The challenges were in particular to take account of the global problems of HIV and its international effects on tuberculosis. They also faced the emerging possibility of incorporating free anti-HIV drugs, previously too expensive for poor countries, into joint treatment facilities. Recent international recommendations updating treating schedules had to be addressed. All these they have tackled with skill and experience, making other modifications to the text where necessary.

In their Preface to this edition they have emphasized the wide global use of the previous editions. Indeed, we estimated that some 100,000 copies in 19 languages have been distributed in many countries throughout the world. I am sure that this outstanding third edition will be equally welcome. The editors will earn the gratitude of many carers and their patients in many countries.

Sir John Crofton
26 February 2008

Preface to the Second Edition

Professor David Morely, the Honorary Director of Teaching Aids at Low Cost (TALC), originally asked the authors to write this book for non-specialist doctors and health professionals in countries with a high prevalence of tuberculosis. We found it a fascinating challenge to try to produce a book in simple language which could be useful to workers who might have very few resources. The book was to be primarily about clinical tuberculosis. But we felt that clinical tuberculosis should be put in a framework of a National Tuberculosis Control Programme. Only in that framework could mass cure lead to mass prevention.

We had hoped that at least some doctors and health professionals in some countries would find the book useful. In the event, the book does seem to have met a real need and demand has exceeded our wildest expectations. We initially arranged for French, Spanish and Portuguese translations, so as to make it available to the appropriate countries in Africa and America. But we have been delighted to find that many countries have wished to produce editions in their own languages. As we write (1997) it has appeared in 14 languages, with editions in four others in various stages of preparation. Besides the languages already mentioned, there are editions in Russian, Italian, Croatian, Chinese, Mongolian, Thai, Vietnamese, Arabic, Farsi (Iran) and Turkish. We are expecting future editions in Romanian, Indonesian, Urdu and Bengali. We are most grateful to the translators, publishers and distributors of all these editions. A preliminary estimate is that more than 70,000 copies in the various languages have been distributed in 125 countries. The book has been used by the World Health Organization (WHO) and the International Union Against Tuberculosis and Lung Disease (IUATLD[a]), and we hope by others, for their training courses.

In producing our first edition we had much help from a series of international experts. These included Professors John Biddulph (Papua New Guinea) and David Morley (TALC and UK); Drs Andrew Cassels (UK), Keith Edwards (Papua New Guinea), A.D. Harries (UK and Malawi), Wendy Holmes (Zimbabwe and Australia), Kanwar K. Kaul (India), A. Kochi (WHO), Colin McDougall (UK), S.J. Nkinda (Ethiopia), Knut Ovreberg (Norway and IUATLD), S.P. Parma (India), C.A. Pearson (UK and Nigeria), Annik Rouillon (France and IUATLD), Sergio Spinaci (WHO), Karel Styblo (Netherlands and IUATLD), H.G. ten Dam (WHO), Yan Bi-Ya (China). Once more we record our gratitude to them.

In preparing this second edition we have benefitted from much discussion with international experts, notably those from WHO and IUATLD. In particular we thank Dr Hans Rieder of IUATLD who reread our first edition in detail and made many helpful suggestions which we have incorporated.

The major changes in the present edition are in the chapters on HIV and tuberculosis and in the sections on chemotherapy. Since the first edition there is now much more experience of HIV. We have greatly expanded that chapter. In doing so we have utilized extensively the WHO publication *TB/HIV. A Clinical*

Manual by Drs A.D. Harries and D. Maher (1996). We are most grateful to Dr Harries for constructive criticism of a draft of our chapter.

We have revised the sections on chemotherapy to make sure that they are consistent with the second (1997) edition of WHO's *Treatment of Tuberculosis. Guidelines for National Programmes.*[b] We have also revised the appendix on tuberculin testing in the light of recent recommendations by the IUATLD and informal discussions with WHO staff.

Much work has been done in recent years on 'molecular' aspects of tuberculosis. The detection of specific components of tubercle bacilli may ultimately lead to rapid diagnosis of disease and to rapid detection of drug resistance. Genetic classification of sub-strains of bacilli can already identify sources of local outbreaks. But none of the new methods is so far sufficiently simple, reliable and cheap for general use in poorer countries. So we have not included any details. The search continues for new drugs but none has yet proved sufficiently effective, non-toxic and cheap to find a place in routine treatment. In all these fields look out for new developments.

Sadly we have to record the death in 1996 of our co-author Fred Miller. He made an outstanding contribution to the book. We hope the book will stand as a memorial to his outstanding work for paediatrics, and in particular paediatric tuberculosis, in many countries. We miss him sorely.

John Crofton
Norman Horne
1999

[a] Now known as The Union.
[b] Note that the WHO updated these treatment guidelines in 2003.

Preface to the First Edition

Professor David Morley, Professor Emeritus of Tropical Child Health, London University, and Honorary Director of Teaching Aids at Low Cost (TALC), asked us to write this book. He thought there was an urgent need for a practical book on clinical tuberculosis for non-specialist doctors and other health professionals working in the many countries where there was still a big tuberculosis problem.

We knew there were already several up-to-date booklets on organizing national tuberculosis control programmes. We therefore asked the International Union Against Tuberculosis and Lung Disease (IUATLD[a]) and the Tuberculosis Unit of the World Health Organization (WHO) in Geneva whether they thought there was a need for a book mainly about the problems of diagnosis and treatment, especially for those working in areas with very few, or only moderate, facilities. They assured us that there was a real need, so we agreed to write the book.

Some of those we have consulted consider that the book would also be useful for doctors in countries now with little tuberculosis. In these countries younger doctors who seldom see such patients may easily miss the diagnosis. They may also have little experience of the practical side of managing the disease.

All three authors had extensive experience with tuberculosis when it was a major problem in the UK and Europe. Between us we have later had much further experience in advising on tuberculosis problems in many countries in Asia, Africa and Latin America, where tuberculosis remains an enormous problem.

This is primarily a book on clinical tuberculosis. But each practising doctor must also play his or her part in the National Tuberculosis Programme, if there is one. We have therefore described the important features of such a programme.

We have attempted to make this a useful and practical guide for the ordinary non-specialized doctor or health professional who will meet tuberculosis in the course of his or her work. We have tried to help with his or her problems, whether working in a district hospital with at least some basic facilities or in an isolated rural area with very few.

We hope that non-medical professionals will also find the book helpful. For those less familiar with the language, we have attempted to keep the English simple.

To be helpful to doctors, we have had to go into some medical detail in certain sections. These sections include the interpretation of X-rays and the often difficult diagnosis of miliary tuberculosis and tuberculous meningitis. But we have separated most of the more difficult medical details of management into a reference section. This will mainly be of concern to doctors.

We wanted to make sure the book was suited to those working in a wide variety of countries. We therefore sent an earlier draft to colleagues on the staffs of the Tuberculosis Unit of the WHO in Geneva and of the IUATLD, as well as other consultants with experience of tuberculosis in Africa, India, China and Papua New Guinea. All gave the book a warm welcome. Most also made useful suggestions.

We have been able to include most of these in the present text. Indeed, as a result, it has been extensively rewritten. Thanks to the help of our colleagues, we believe that the book now presents much collective wisdom. We are deeply grateful to all these experts for taking so much time and trouble to make the book as good as possible. We record our heartfelt thanks to the following:

Professor John Biddulph, Professor of Child Health, University of Papua New Guinea; Senior Paediatrician, Health Department, Papua New Guinea

Dr Andrew Cassels, Liverpool School of Tropical Medicine, UK; former Medical Director, Britain Nepal Medical Trust

Dr Keith Edwards, Senior Lecturer in Child Health, University of Papua New Guinea

Dr Wendy Holmes, formerly Government Medical Officer, Chinhoyi Provincial Hospital, Zimbabwe; at present Medical Officer, Victoria Aboriginal Health Service, Australia

Dr Kanwar K. Kaul, Professor of Paediatrics, Jabalpur, India

Dr A. Kochi, Chief Medical Officer, Tuberculosis Unit, WHO, Geneva

Dr Colin McDougall, former Leprosy Consultant to the Ministry of Health, Lusaka, Zambia; Consultant in Clinical Research (Leprosy) to the British Leprosy Relief Association (LEPRA): Editor of *Leprosy Review*

Professor David Morley, Professor Emeritus of Tropical Child Health, University of London; Honorary Director, TALC

Dr S. J. Nkinda, Director of Training, All Africa Leprosy and Rehabilitation Training Centre, Addis Ababa, Ethiopia; responsible for IUATLD Training Courses for Africa

Dr Knut Ovreberg, Chairman, Project Advisory Group, IUATLD

Dr S. P. Parma, formerly Director, New Delhi Tuberculosis Centre; Chairman of Technical Committee and Honorary Technical Advisor, Tuberculosis Association of India; Chairman, Tuberculosis Expert Group, Indian Council of Medical Research

Dr Annik Rouillon, Executive Director, IUATLD

Dr Sergio Spinaci, Tuberculosis Unit, WHO, Geneva

Dr Karel Styblo, Director of Scientific Activities, IUATLD; Director Tuberculosis Surveillance Research Unit, The Hague, the Netherlands

Mr H. G. ten Dam, Tuberculosis Unit, WHO, Geneva

Dr Yan Bi-Ya, Director, Beijing Research Unit, People's Republic of China

Further thanks are also due. Dr Keith Edwards, Dr Wendy Holmes, Dr G. J. Ebrahim and Professor David Morely permitted us to include some of their own original material; we acknowledge these at appropriate points in the text. Dr A.D. Harries of the Liverpool School of Tropical Medicine advised us on the management of severe drug reactions in patients with HIV infection and tuberculosis. Dr C.A. Pearson, with long experience in Nigeria, drew our attention to hypomelanosis (decreased pigmentation) in African patients with tuberculosis.

Many people have helped us with the production of this book. We are most grateful to Mr Ian Lennox of the Medical Illustration Department, Edinburgh University, for turning our amateur sketches into clear and intelligible drawings. We thank our secretaries Mss Elizabeth Ann Pretty, Joyce Holywell and Sharon White for preparing initial drafts. Further and particular thanks are due to Mrs E.A. Pretty for word-processing revision after revision of successive draft texts, and for handling a complex series of tasks with unfailing enthusiasm and intelligence.

We thank Mrs Fiona Swann-Skimming and the Chest, Heart and Stroke Association, Scotland, for producing numerous photocopies of an earlier text for despatch to our consultant advisors worldwide.

We are deeply grateful to Mr Rex Parry and Mrs Sheila Jones of Macmillan Education Ltd for so skilfully nursing us through the ups and downs of publication. It was a real pleasure to work with professionals so understanding of what we were trying to do and so enthusiastic about helping us to do it.

A top priority for TALC, IUATLD, authors and publishers has been to make the book both cheaply and widely available in countries with a major tuberculosis problem. This has required substantial financial help to underpin the costs of publication and distribution. We are very grateful indeed to a number of organizations for generous donations in support of these costs.

We give our warmest thanks to Dr Annik Rouillon, Executive Director, and Dr Karel Styblo, Director of Scientific Activities, of IUATLD for their unstinting help and support. The book is formally sponsored by both The Union and by TALC. Indeed, as indicated above, it would not have been written without the initiative and enthusiasm of Professor David Morley, TALC's Honorary Director. His organization exports over 50,000 books annually to poorer countries. Professor Morley also made many helpful suggestions during the writing of the book.

We also warmly thank Dr A. Kochi, Dr Sergio Spinaci and Mr H.G. ten Dam of WHO's Tuberculosis Unit in Geneva, not only for their constructive comments on an earlier text, as listed above, but for much personal encouragement and advice.

J. Crofton
N. Horne
F. Miller
1992

[a] Now known as The Union.

Foreword to the First Edition

The International Union Against Tuberculosis and Lung Disease welcomes *Clinical Tuberculosis* with interest, gratitude and pride.

Interest, because clinical aspects are part and parcel of the essential knowledge necessary both to those dealing with the individual and those dealing with the community.

Gratitude, because precisely this type of manual for non-specialized practitioners and public health field workers was long and badly needed.

Pride, because the book is the result of the collaborative effort of two long-standing highly respected members of the Union, and a paediatrician, all of them with an immense experience with tuberculosis patients as well as with the problems and needs at national and international levels. The book bears witness to their indefatigable drive in trying to impart useful know-how to their colleagues and fellow workers striving under difficult conditions.

We now possess well-established methods for the prevention, diagnosis and treatment of tuberculosis, as well as the concept of the National Tuberculosis Programmes; the latter provide the system though which the effective means can be delivered.

Recent studies have re-awakened our awareness as to the magnitude of the problem: tuberculosis remains the biggest killer in the world as a single pathogen; while it hits children as well as the elderly, the worst affected are adults between 15 and 59 years of age i.e. the parents, workers and leaders of society. Tuberculosis accounts for 26% of all avoidable deaths in Third World countries.

The tremendous toll of tuberculosis is increasing in many countries due to the interaction with HIV and tuberculosis infections. However, tuberculosis remains curable even in the HIV infected. The present remobilization against the ancient scourge of tuberculosis will, hopefully, be able to curb the present flaring up of incidence.

Moreover, cost–benefit analyses have shown that short-course chemotherapy of tuberculosis, within the framework of national programmes, is one of the cheapest of all health interventions, comparable in cost to immunization for measles or to oral rehydration therapy for diarrhoea.

Those who fight tuberculosis, this inseparable but terrible companion of man, will find this comprehensive and clear book a mighty ally to assist them accomplish their mission with more competence, more understanding and more humanity, and will bring closer the time when proper diagnosis and adequate management of cases will stop the perpetuation of the disease, thus paving the way to its elimination.

Annik Rouillon, MD, MPH
Executive Director
International Union Against
Tuberculosis and Lung Disease
1992

[a] Now known as The Union.

Abbreviations

The editors of this book have largely avoided using abbreviations, with the following exceptions.

TB   **Tubercle bacilli:** this commonly refers to *Mycobacterium tuberculosis*, but it may also be used for *M. bovis* (the organism that causes tuberculosis in cattle, from which it can be transmitted to humans), and *M. africanum*, a variant between *M. tuberculosis* and *M. bovis*, that is found among some patients in Africa and in some other areas of the world. Microscopic examination identifies 'acid-fast bacilli', not tubercle bacilli (other mycobacteria are also acid-fast, and some other bacteria may also be acid-fast). In the practice of national tuberculosis programmes, a microscopy result 'positive for acid-fast bacilli' is almost always the same as TB and the clinician must always treat it as such. For simplicity, we will thus also use 'TB' for the microscopy finding of acid-fast bacilli.

HIV   **Human immunodeficiency virus:** a virus that destroys the immune function among persons infected with it, with the result that HIV-infected persons get many diseases more frequently than they would if they weren't infected by it.

AIDS   **Acquired immunodeficiency syndrome:** a patient with advanced HIV infection is said to have AIDS when serious illnesses become manifest.

Chapter 1
General background to clinical tuberculosis

.1 Introduction

About this book

This book is written for non-specialist hospital doctors, doctors in primary health care and other health professionals who may meet tuberculosis in the course of their work. Almost all patients with newly diagnosed tuberculosis can be cured if properly treated. Many will die if they are not properly treated. As a responsible doctor or health worker, therefore:

▶ do not miss the diagnosis
▶ do then give the correct treatment for the full period of time.

More than that, good treatment is the most important form of prevention because it makes infectious patients non-infectious. This reduces the chance that the infection will be passed on in the community.

Tuberculosis is a challenging disease. Sometimes trying to make the diagnosis is like trying to solve a detective story. But if you succeed, you can be sure of a happy ending to the story in most cases. Modern treatment is highly successful in curing tuberculosis, even in patients already infected with human immunodeficiency virus (HIV), the virus that causes the acquired immunodeficiency syndrome (AIDS).

Some things you should know

If you are going to play your part in helping your patients, and in dealing with tuberculosis in your country, you must know something about its cause. You must know where infection comes from. You must understand that most people who have that infection do not get ill, and why some do develop the disease. The general public will also expect you to know something about the best way of preventing tuberculosis. Your country has a national programme for tuberculosis control, and you should know about it and should play your part in making it work.

The worldwide problem of tuberculosis

In many industrialized countries, money, other resources, rising standards of living and widespread use of medications to treat tuberculosis in the last 50 years have helped to reduce the disease so that it affects only small numbers of people. But in poorer countries tuberculosis remains as big a problem as ever. Indeed, because of increases in populations and the spread of HIV infection, there are probably more tuberculosis patients in the world today than ever before. The World

Health Organization (WHO) estimated that the total number of new tuberculosis cases in the world was 8.9 million in 2004 (140 per 100 000 population), of whom 3.9 million were smear-positive (62 per 100 000 population). An estimated 1.7 million people died from tuberculosis in 2004. These trends could be reversed if most countries implemented National Tuberculosis Programmes effectively, along with National AIDS Programmes to control HIV infection.

The outlook

This may all sound depressing; however, in many poor countries with high tuberculosis rates, modern programmes, efficiently applied, are showing excellent results. There are even signs that this success is beginning to make tuberculosis a little less frequent in some of these countries where rates of HIV infection are low. In industrialized countries the rate of new cases (notification rate of new cases) fell by 6–12% a year after the widespread use of drug treatment. After the introduction of good national programmes, the WHO reported declines per year of 5% for Chile, 7% for Cuba, 8% for Uruguay and 7% for the Republic of Korea. These figures show what can be achieved. But with the explosion of HIV infection in sub-Saharan Africa, and now in some countries of eastern Europe, the former Soviet Union and Asia, a truly major national and international effort will be needed to achieve such results throughout the world. An increasing number of countries have made a good start. We hope you will make your own contribution in your own country.

1.2 General guidelines on the treatment of tuberculosis

In many countries some doctors give poor or inadequate treatment. This is likely:
▶ to fail to cure the patient
▶ to leave them with drug-resistant tubercle bacilli (TB), making it difficult for anyone else to cure them
▶ to leave them alive (at least for some time) and infectious, perhaps with drug-resistant bacilli, so that they spread the disease to others.

So poor treatment is both poor doctoring and poor public health.

Here we provide some general guidelines and 'dos and don'ts' that will help to avoid common errors. We suggest you read these first, though we realize that you may not need this basic advice. Then go on (or refer when necessary) to the later parts of this book that give more detail.

Dos and don'ts for doctors

Don'ts
Avoid the following errors, which are common in some countries.
1 Never treat a patient with probable pulmonary tuberculosis without examining the sputum. (An exception to this rule is small children, who often have no sputum; diagnosis may have to be largely clinical in these cases.)

2 Never give a single drug alone: drug resistance usually follows and is permanent.

3 Never add a single drug to a drug combination if the patient becomes worse. First, make sure that the patient is taking the drug combination regularly. If they are but are still getting worse, the bacilli may well be resistant to all the drugs being used. Adding one drug is the same as giving one drug alone. The patient's TB will soon be resistant to this also.

4 Never fail to follow up the patient and make sure that the full recommended course of treatment has been taken. It is important to make sure that someone sees the patient taking every dose whenever rifampicin is used.

5 Never use a combination of streptomycin and penicillin for non-tuberculous conditions. It is seldom better than penicillin alone or tetracycline and may induce streptomycin resistance if the patient has undiagnosed tuberculosis. Rifampicin should *only* be used to treat tuberculosis or leprosy.

6 Never use a fluoroquinolone in the treatment of pneumonia without excluding the possibility of tuberculosis.

7 Never treat only on the advice of representatives of drug companies. Their advice will be prejudiced and may well be wrong.

Dos

Remember the following important and simple rules.

1 Always examine the sputum in a suspected case. It is the only certain method of diagnosis. If sputum is negative, but X-ray is suggestive, give antibiotics first and repeat sputum examinations if the patient remains symptomatic: it may be transient pneumonia (or lung abscess).

2 Only use recommended drug combinations. It is dangerous to use drug combinations that have not been proved, or are known to be bad or risky; virtually all patients can be cured by established methods.

3 It is vital to convince the patient (and his or her family) that he or she must complete the full course of treatment (6 or 8 months with combinations containing rifampicin and pyrazinamide) to avoid relapse. Explanatory leaflets are useful and should be available in your country. Even with illiterate patients, someone in the family or village can read the leaflet.

4 It is essential to be kind and sympathetic to the patient. Patients are much more likely to come back and to complete treatment if they believe you are their friend and that you want to help them personally.

5 Remember that if a patient has completed a course of treatment and relapsed, or has missed two or more consecutive months of treatment and returns with positive sputum, or remains sputum positive after 5 months of treatment, you should give the patient a (different) standard retreatment regimen.

6 If a patient has had several courses of previous treatment (perhaps with poor drug combinations) and has now relapsed, refer to a specialist (or obtain advice in writing). Planning treatment in such cases is difficult and a mistake

can be fatal. Your National Tuberculosis Programme may have a special drug regimen for such patients.

Cautions

Details of recommended drug regimens are given in Chapter 6. Remember the following important points.

1 Most apparent failures to respond to treatment are because treatment duration has been too short. This is usually because the doctor or patient doesn't realize the importance of completing a full course with no interruptions. This is much more likely to happen if directly observed therapy was not carried out.

   Unfortunately another reason could be that a member of staff has stolen drugs instead of giving them to the patient. Yet another reason may be that the patient has sold the drugs instead of swallowing them!

   Other failures are due to bad or irregular treatment with poor drug combinations: a poorly trained doctor or health assistant may have prescribed bad treatment; or may have failed to instruct the patient about what pills to take, when to take them and the importance of taking them regularly. In this case the patient's TB may have developed drug resistance.

2 Patients who have not taken a first-line recommended regimen for as much as 1 month are likely to have TB that are still susceptible (sensitive) to standard drugs. They can safely be put on a first-line regimen.

3 If you are using a rifampicin-containing regimen:
   ▶ Make sure the patient can take drugs regularly by being directly observed to swallow them.
   ▶ Give one of the recommended drug regimens. Other regimens may result in failure, the development of resistant TB or early relapse.

Guidelines for health staff other than doctors

As a health worker you should ensure that all your staff know and act on the following summary.

Tuberculosis can be cured.
THE PATIENT'S LIFE DEPENDS ON YOU.

Tuberculosis is an infectious disease, spread mainly through cough. Thus, *everyone* should cover their mouth when coughing.

If a patient has any of the following, consider him or her a 'tuberculosis suspect':
▶ cough for 3 or more weeks
▶ coughing up blood-stained sputum or, in serious cases, blood

▶ pain in the chest for 3 or more weeks
▶ fever for 3 or more weeks.

All these can be due to other diseases, but sputum must be tested if any of these symptoms are present.

Sputum examination is much more reliable than X-ray. If two (or three) sputum samples are negative, give simple treatment (not anti-tuberculosis drugs) but repeat sputum examination if symptoms continue, and/or refer the patient to a tuberculosis clinic or a doctor. Diagnosis in children can be difficult. If possible refer to a doctor.

If sputum is positive, tuberculosis can be easily cured if the patient takes the full course of treatment.

Symptoms soon clear but treatment must continue regularly for the full period recommended. Otherwise tuberculosis comes back and treatment has to start all over again.

BCG is a good protection against tuberculosis in children, especially against the fatal forms of tuberculous meningitis and miliary tuberculosis.

Dos and *don'ts* in tuberculosis

- DO always examine the sputum when there are symptoms suggestive of possible tuberculosis.
- DO make sure that the patient understands the need for a full period of treatment, even though symptoms will soon clear. Give the patient a leaflet on treatment, if available.
- DO explain this to the patient's relatives.
- DO be kind and sympathetic: then the patient is more likely to come back regularly for treatment. Think of the patient as a friend you want to help.
- DO examine all family/home contacts, especially if they are ill.
- DO put the patient's name in the tuberculosis register and give a treatment card with each date of attendance. Make sure the patient understands and remembers the dates.
- DO send someone to visit the home if the patient fails to come for any appointment. A letter is usually not sufficient.
- DO check your supplies of anti-tuberculosis drugs frequently and see that you don't run out.
- DON'T forget that anyone with a chronic cough may have tuberculosis, especially if there is also fever and loss of weight.
- DON'T forget to test the sputum.
- DON'T forget to follow up patients who fail to come back and persuade them to complete treatment.

> # Tuberculosis can be cured.
> # You can do more than anyone else
> # to save the patient's life.

1.3 The battle between TB and the patient

Causes of tuberculosis: the bacillus

The human tubercle bacillus (*Mycobacterium tuberculosis*) is the main cause of tuberculosis all over the world.

A slightly different type of TB, *Mycobacterium africanum,* occurs in Africa. The only important difference is that it is often resistant to thioacetazone.

The bovine bacillus (*Mycobacterium bovis*) at one time caused much infection in cattle in Europe and the Americas. Infection was often passed on to man through contaminated milk. Bovine TB in milk can be killed by boiling the milk, and bovine tuberculosis rarely occurs where this is the practice. The extent of the transmission of bovine tuberculosis to humans is difficult to determine because of technical problems in isolating the organisms. One important difference is the resistance to pyrazinamide in *M. bovis*.

Environmental mycobacteria (sometimes also called non-tuberculous mycobacteria, atypical mycobacteria, or mycobacteria other than tubercle bacilli) include a wide range of bacterial species. Most are harmless, provided the affected individual has a well-functioning immune system. They are common in the environments of many countries where tuberculosis is also frequent but they seldom cause disease in those whose immune system functions well. When the immune system is suppressed (such as in persons living with HIV/AIDS), these infections can be lethal. Nevertheless, harmless infection in humans can give rise to a weakly positive tuberculin skin test. (Disease from these bacilli has become relatively more important in some developed countries, such as parts of the USA, Europe and Australia, where ordinary tuberculosis has now greatly decreased. It may also develop in patients infected with HIV. As these bacilli are resistant to most commonly used drugs, the disease is more difficult to treat.)

Nearly all tuberculosis in countries with a high burden of the disease is caused by the common TB, *M. tuberculosis*, so that is what most of this book is about.

Infection and disease

In the past, when tuberculosis was widespread in industrialized countries, it was possible to show by skin-testing with tuberculin that most young adults had become infected. But only a small proportion (about 10%) developed the disease. This is still what happens in most countries where tuberculosis is a problem and HIV is not a major problem.

Whether infection goes on to disease *(Figure 1.1)* depends mainly on the *defences* of the person infected (host resistance).

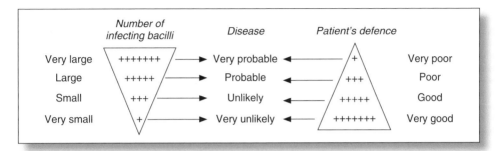

Figure 1.1 *Probability of developing tuberculosis.* The influence of the number of bacilli (exposure) and the strength of the patient's defences on the risk of developing tuberculosis following infection.

In some cases, infection may rapidly go on to disease. In others, TB may remain 'dormant', with a few 'sleeping' bacilli kept under control by the defences, but some later lowering of the patient's defences (e.g. by malnutrition, by another disease (such as HIV infection) or just old age) may allow the dormant TB to multiply and cause disease *(Figure 1.2)*. In most people, their host defences either kill off all the bacilli or, perhaps more often, keep them suppressed and under long-term control.

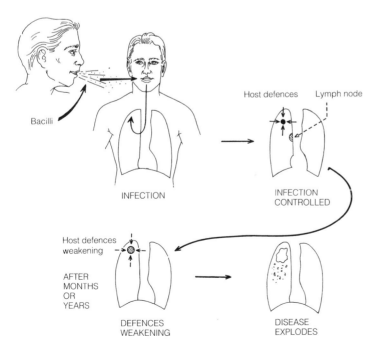

Figure 1.2
Tuberculosis infection and the host's (patient's) defences. At first the patient's defences may keep the TB under control. After months or years, the infected person's defences may weaken (e.g. from malnutrition or another disease). Then the disease starts to spread in the lung. A cavity may develop in the lung. The sputum may become positive for TB and the patient may infect children and other people.

Sources of infection – where it comes from

Tuberculosis in the lung is by far the most important source. Coughing and talking produce very small droplets that contain TB. They are so small that they float in the air. These may be inhaled and cause infection and then disease.

Patients with positive sputum on direct smear (i.e. TB visible under the microscope) are much more infectious, because they are producing far more TB, than those positive only on culture (therefore, you can see them clearly under the microscope). The closer someone is to the patient and the longer the two live together, the higher the chance that the person in contact with the patient will inhale TB. An infant of an infectious mother will be at particular risk. It is important to teach infectious patients to cover their mouths and to turn their faces away when they cough. This becomes less important after 2–3 weeks of treatment (see below) if the patient has disease caused by bacilli that are susceptible to the medications.

Chemotherapy rapidly reduces infectiousness, usually within 2 weeks, if the bacilli are susceptible. This is why good treatment of all tuberculosis patients, and particularly patients with a direct positive sputum smear, is by far the most effective method of prevention. But if treatment is not continued for the full period, the patient may develop disease again and become infectious again.

Urine and discharges from tuberculosis patients are usually not infectious because they do not form tiny droplets that can float in the air, and they contain relatively few bacilli.

Children with tuberculosis are usually not infectious, because they do not cough out TB (their sputum smears are negative). If they do have positive smears, however, they are just as infectious as adults.

Lessons for prevention

In prevention, your most important priority as a doctor is therefore to diagnose patients with a direct positive sputum smear and to make sure that they complete a standardized treatment. These sputum-smear-positive patients are also usually the most ill. They need treatment urgently to save their lives.

Sterilization of sputum, bedclothes, etc.

▶ Direct sunlight kills TB very quickly. Exposure to sunlight is therefore a convenient method in sunny climates. (But bacilli may survive for years in the dark: much spread of infection probably occurs in dark houses or huts.)
▶ Sodium hypochlorite (household bleach) liquefies sputum and kills TB but has to be used in glass jars as it damages metal. It also bleaches dyed material if dropped on it. Add to the sputum twice its volume of 1% hypochlorite. (Note that TB may resist 5% phenol for several hours.)
▶ Heat: TB are destroyed in 20 minutes at 60°C and in 5 minutes at 70°C.
▶ Paper handkerchiefs should be burnt as soon as possible after use. (Old newspapers or other similar material can also be used and then burnt.)

▶ Exposure to air and sunlight is a good and simple method, particularly in sunny climates, for dealing with blankets, clothes or materials.

Environmental hygiene

The aim is to reduce the risk from undiagnosed infectious patients. There is a limit to what can be achieved in poorer countries but the following could help.

▶ *Reduce overcrowding* wherever possible (which also reduces other infectious respiratory diseases, such as pneumonia in infants).
▶ *Improve ventilation* of houses.
▶ *Discourage smoking* in public places. Smoking increases the risk of tuberculosis.

Host defences – how a person resists infection

Many things affect the way our bodies fight TB.

Age and sex

Up to 2 years of age, infection is particularly liable to result in the most fatal forms, miliary tuberculosis and tuberculous meningitis, due to bloodstream spread. Infants and young children of both sexes have weak defences. After 2 years of age, and before puberty, an infected child may develop disseminated disease or meningitis, or one of the extra-pulmonary forms, particularly lymph node, bone or joint disease. Before puberty, the lung part of the primary lesion usually just affects that local area, though cavities like those in adults may be seen, especially in children with severe malnutrition and girls aged 10–14 years. The lymph node part of the primary complex may also give rise to lung collapse and other complications. There is little difference between boys and girls up to puberty.

When tuberculosis was common in industrialized countries, the peak incidence of pulmonary tuberculosis was usually in young adults. The rate continued fairly high at all ages in men, but in women the rate dropped rapidly after the childbearing years. Women often developed pulmonary tuberculosis following childbirth. As the frequency of disease declined, the age of tuberculosis patients increased. Pulmonary tuberculosis cases occurred more frequently in older age groups in both sexes but were more common in men than in women, largely due to the fact that older people had a much higher likelihood of having been infected at some point in their lives.

Nutrition

Starvation or malnutrition reduces resistance to the disease. This is a very important factor in poorer communities, in both adults and children.

Drug-induced immunosuppression

Immunosuppressant treatments used for treating certain diseases such as cancer also increase the chance of developing tuberculosis.

Poverty

This leads to poor-quality and overcrowded housing or poor work conditions. These may lower defences as well as making infection more likely. People living in such conditions are often also poorly nourished. The whole complex of poverty makes it easier for the TB to cause disease.

Lessons for prevention

Many of the factors we have been describing can only be removed by economic development or government action to decrease poverty and improve nutrition. In industrialized countries this has been perhaps the most important factor in the long-term decrease of tuberculosis over the last century. As a doctor, you may not be able to do much about this. But in recent years large-scale effective treatment has speeded up the decline in tuberculosis by reducing the numbers of infectious people in the population. You can – and must – contribute to this in your own area. The priority is to identify sputum-smear-positive patients in a timely manner and to make sure that they all complete effective treatment.

Reducing national tobacco consumption will help to prevent tuberculosis, as well as preventing lung (and other) cancers, coronary heart disease, chronic bronchitis, and a host of other conditions. As a doctor, and a leader of opinion, you can do a lot about this. In particular, do not smoke yourself, and certainly never in front of patients.

BCG vaccination

BCG is a vaccine consisting of live bacilli which have lost their power to cause disease (except in persons with profound immunodeficiency). The bacilli originally came from a strain of bovine TB grown for many years in the laboratory. BCG stimulates immunity, increasing the body's defences without itself causing damage. Following BCG vaccination, in most cases the body's increased defences will control or kill any TB that enter the body.

Some controlled trials have shown that BCG can provide up to 80% protection against tuberculosis for as long as 10 years if administered before first infection (i.e. to tuberculin-negative children). However, other large trials have failed to show benefit in reducing tuberculosis overall. Most trials in infants in poor countries have shown important protection against disseminated tuberculosis and tuberculous meningitis.

The current recommendation by the WHO and the International Union Against Tuberculosis and Lung Disease (The Union) is that in countries with high prevalence of tuberculosis, BCG should be given routinely to all infants (but with a few exceptions, such as those known to have HIV infection and children of mothers with HIV infection at high risk of TB transmission). The normal dose in neonates and infants is 0.05 ml.

The effect of BCG probably lasts 10–15 years. However, no trial has yet shown any benefit of repeating BCG vaccination.

Because the main effect of infant vaccination is to protect children, and because children with primary tuberculosis are not usually infectious, BCG has little effect in reducing the number of infectious cases in the population. To reduce these it is much more important to give good treatment to all sputum-smear-positive patients. Of course we should give BCG routinely to all infants as a protection in childhood.

1.4 National Tuberculosis Programmes

Most countries where tuberculosis is a significant problem now have national programmes for tuberculosis *(Table 1.1)*. Some of the items in this table are essential components of the WHO's 'Stop TB Strategy'.

In some countries the programme is combined with the Leprosy Programme. It is important that you play your part in the national programme in your country. It is poor doctoring to be ignorant of the programme and even worse to know about it and not to do your best to carry it out in your own work.

Table 1.1 Essentials of tuberculosis control programmes
1 National and local agreement to have a programme
2 National and local health education about tuberculosis
3 Case finding by routine sputum microscopy for TB in those with symptoms
4 Standard supervised treatment
5 Methods for recalling defaulters
6 Standard records and monitoring
7 Ensuring uninterrupted supply of drugs and other supplies
8 Regular training and retraining
9 BCG vaccination of the newborn
10 Examination of family contacts

With the increase in HIV infection in some countries, national programmes will have to take account of this in both diagnosis and treatment.

The aim of a national programme is to use limited resources to prevent, diagnose and treat the disease in the best and most effective way.

The programme is most likely to succeed if it has been fully discussed by representatives of all those who will take part in it. This includes central, intermediate (regional, provincial) and district administrators; specialist and general doctors, nurses and health workers from institutes, laboratories, hospitals and primary care; representatives of both health and finance ministries; and representatives, politicians and others of the general population and local communities.

After agreement among all these groups at a central level, it is important to hold seminars in different parts of the country at local level and to involve health care facilities at all levels. It is important that representatives of the local population be consulted so that arrangements can fit in with local customs and convenience. Health workers must find out the local beliefs about tuberculosis, so that education about the disease and its treatment can be adapted to those beliefs.

Note on local beliefs

Local beliefs about tuberculosis and its cause will obviously vary between countries, areas, cultures and even different groups of the population in the same area. Religion, social class, ethnic group and level of education may influence peoples' ideas. In some places, people believe that tuberculosis is due to evil spirits that have got into the patient. Even where people know that tuberculosis is an infectious disease, they may think a particular person has got the disease by being bewitched. In one area, most ordinary people thought that a patient usually caught tuberculosis from the stick that was used for cleaning the teeth. In another, people thought that the symptoms were often due to a sin such as adultery. Information, education and communication activities should address these local beliefs.

You may be able to persuade local healers to send patients with possible tuberculosis to health centres for diagnosis and treatment. Explain to them that if they try to treat these patients themselves they will fail. This will be bad for their local reputation and their practice.

In many cultures people think that tuberculosis is hereditary. This idea is not surprising. Tuberculosis is an infectious disease. Often several members of the family, sometimes in different generations, may develop it. Unfortunately this idea often means that people are ashamed of the disease. They feel that it is a disgrace to the family. If a daughter gets tuberculosis, the family may be afraid that they will never find her a husband. This idea may remain even after she is obviously cured. If this is a common misconception in the community in which you work, try to educate opinion leaders so that patients and their families do not suffer from this additional anxiety. In our experience, the idea disappears when the community realizes that good treatment is easily available and almost always cures the disease. Cured patients may be able to help in educating both new patients and the community.

If your country has a National Tuberculosis Programme make sure that you and your staff know its details and help to make it successful.

Components of a National Tuberculosis Programme

The model National Tuberculosis Programme (Table 1.1)
Details of model national programmes are given in: *Management of Tuberculosis. A Guide for the Essentials of Good Practice,* 6th edn, due to be published by The Union in 2009. We give a brief outline here.

Case finding

▶ Examine the sputum of all patients who have had a cough and sputum for 3 weeks or longer. (Cough due to an acute infection will usually be clearing up, or will have gone, by 3 weeks. Cough due to tuberculosis will be unchanged or getting worse.) This is particularly important if the patient has also lost weight, has fever or pain in the chest or has coughed up blood (*Figure 1.3*). Some patients have these last symptoms without any chronic cough. Regard any patient who has any of these symptoms as a 'tuberculosis suspect' and examine the sputum for TB.

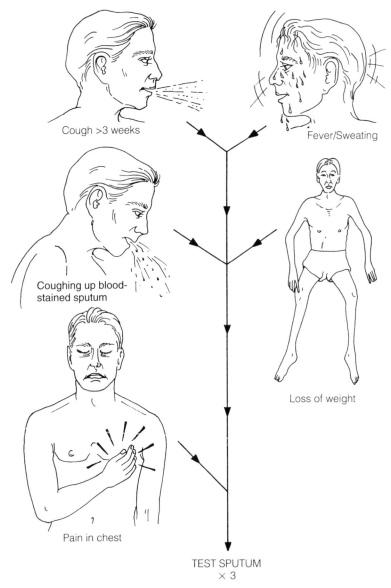

Figure 1.3 *Diagnosing pulmonary tuberculosis.* The most important symptoms.

▶ Investigate and follow up any patient with a chest X-ray showing a shadow. In particular, examine the sputum for TB. Indiscriminate X-ray of the whole population is, however, expensive and unreliable and we do not recommend it. Sputum testing of tuberculosis suspects is much more reliable.

▶ The terms 'active' and 'passive' case finding are used to describe whether health workers go to the community to find the patients (active) or patients come to health facilities because of other symptoms (passive). Most patients with tuberculosis who are ill will attend some health care facility (health centre, hospital, out-patient clinic or private doctor), but will be diagnosed only if there is a policy that the sputum of all suspects presenting to a health care facility is routinely examined for TB. This is 'passive case finding', which is conscientiously identifying those with chronic chest symptoms (suspects) among those presenting themselves to health facilities and ensuring that they have sputum smear examination. Many cases are missed because they are not recognized by the health service and do not have sputum smear examination when they come to the service with symptoms. Passive case finding is highly cost-effective, provided it is done properly: it is the standard method in the majority of national programmes. 'Active case finding' involves going to peoples' homes or workplaces and asking them to produce sputum for testing or, as done in the past in many countries, screening them using chest X-ray. This is very expensive and gives far fewer positives. The exception to this general rule on active case finding is household examination.

▶ It is important to help the poor to overcome their limited access to health services. If people in the community know that patients with tuberculosis in their area get good treatment from understanding and friendly health workers, and are cured, then far more people come looking for help. Only when patients who come with symptoms are properly tested, treated and cured is it appropriate to refocus efforts to targeting high-risk groups.

Diagnosis

▶ Microscopy of the sputum is by far the most reliable (and the most accessible) method that you can use, and it can be done almost anywhere. If you have the laboratory resources, try to have at least two specimens examined from each patient.

▶ Because chronic cough may be due to smoking, asthma or chronic bronchitis, many specimens of sputum will be negative. You must test *all* patients with chronic cough, especially those with weight loss or other symptoms that might be due to tuberculosis. Do this wherever you work: in primary care clinic, hospital or private practice. Not to do this is bad medicine.

▶ Tuberculosis is difficult to diagnose with certainty from a chest X-ray alone. Never treat such a patient without having examined the sputum. X-rays are expensive, especially for the poor. Patients are often treated unnecessarily for tuberculosis that they do not have (they may be 'overdiagnosed'). Always have the results of sputum examinations before you make any clinical decision to start anti-tuberculosis treatment. X-rays are needed for smear-negative suspects who remain symptomatic after a course of antibiotics, in particular for tuberculosis suspects who are HIV-positive.

▶ Tuberculin tests are rarely available in poor countries. Where available, test results are also difficult to interpret. But a strongly positive test in a child suspected of tuberculosis can be helpful.

Laboratory services

▶ Microscopy is the most important means of diagnosis and must be made widely available. With a population of 50 000–150 000 it requires proper decentralization to a community level. It must be well supervised to ensure quality.

▶ Culture for TB may be introduced later as services develop. It is most often used for drug-resistance surveys. Culture helps to improve the accuracy of diagnosis in cases that are negative on microscopy.

▶ Testing for drug resistance is expensive for routine use, the results come very late, and are often not reliable if quality assurance is lacking. It is desirable to have a national reference laboratory that can monitor drug-resistance trends in a sample of patients, so that the authorities can understand the problem and take necessary actions.

Standard treatment for new cases of tuberculosis

▶ The WHO and The Union recommend short-course chemotherapy containing rifampicin at least in the intensive phase. These regimens last 6–8 months.

▶ For patients who relapse, who return after default, or who are identified as having failed to respond to standard treatment, the WHO recommends one of the retreatment regimens outlined in Section A.4 (page 158). This will be effective in most such patients. Whenever directly observed treatment is not strictly practised, failure to respond is more likely to be due to not having taken full treatment, rather than to drug resistance. The retreatment regimen will be effective when there is resistance to only one or two drugs (but not to both isoniazid and rifampicin, termed 'multidrug resistance'). 'Chronic cases' who have had repeated poor treatment are more likely to have multidrug-resistant TB.

Treatment supervision

The policy regarding supervision is the responsibility of the National Programme. The whole success of the Programme depends on good supervision of treatment. Treatment should be directly observed (i.e. the patient should be seen to swallow each dose) whenever rifampicin is used. In order to encourage regular attendance, make sure the patient is not kept waiting. In some remote areas, methods for directly observed treatment may have to be adapted; this is the responsibility of the Programme to define. The Programme also spells out the method for recalling patients who have failed to report for treatment ('late patient tracing').

Records

In order to run a successful Tuberculosis Programme there must be good records.

▶ Records are important for you in your *clinic/health centre* so that you can make sure that you fully follow up your patients and that all patients complete treatment.

▶ Reports from clinics/health centres are important at *district/area* level so that administrators can make sure you have the drugs and materials you need to diagnose and treat your patients. They can also compare the work of different clinics and compare their own results with those of other districts.

▶ Reports from districts are important at *national* level for evaluating programme implementation, comparing districts and planning supplies.

▶ Filling in forms may be regarded as a nuisance but, as with all well-managed public health activities, it is an essential part of the proper care of any patient and of a good National Tuberculosis Programme. Make sure you and your staff do it carefully and well. It is important for your own day-to-day work in ensuring that nothing is missed in the care of your patient. It is also an important step to getting the materials and support you need for your patients.

▶ The Programme determines the methods for recording numbers of patients with sputum samples tested, numbers found positive, routine follow-up of patients with regular sputum tests to evaluate sputum conversion to negative, and outcome of treatment. The easiest way to collect relevant information on case finding and evaluation of treatment is to have a 'tuberculosis case register' in every tuberculosis management unit. This should contain each patient's name, address, site of disease, whether the sputum smear was positive on diagnosis, and results of smear examinations at follow-up until treatment is completed. In countries with a high prevalence of HIV, it may contain information concerning testing and care for HIV infection.

▶ This record will give an indication of how enthusiastically health workers are looking for patients and how successful they are in curing them with a full course of treatment.

The Programme may define the type of patient to be recorded.

New patients

▶ Smear-positive pulmonary tuberculosis: at least one positive direct sputum smear.

▶ Culture-positive pulmonary tuberculosis: in areas where culture is possible.

▶ Smear-negative pulmonary tuberculosis: diagnosis made on clinical grounds and/or X-ray: normally this diagnosis should only be made by a doctor.

▶ Extra-pulmonary tuberculosis: confirmed by bacteriology or histology. Clinical diagnosis, usually by a doctor: diagnosis will include organ affected (e.g. lymph node tuberculosis, tuberculous meningitis, spinal tuberculosis).

Retreatment patients: including treatment after relapse, after default and after failure
▶ *Treatment after relapse:* Patients who have previously been cured and now return with bacteriological evidence (e.g. positive sputum smear) of active tuberculosis.
▶ *Treatment after failure:* a new patient who is still sputum smear positive 5 months or more after starting standard treatment. (This is more often due to failure to take a full course of treatment, particularly if the patient was not strictly observed in taking medications, than to drug resistance.)
▶ *Treatment after default:* Patients who have interrupted treatment for 2 or more months and returned with a positive sputum smear.
▶ *Transfers in:* Patients who are transferred from another institution or practice to continue the treatment already started.

Record forms and registers
Your National Programme will provide these.

All these will build up a picture of national progress in case finding and treatment. They will also show up local differences, which may be due to differences in either the amount of tuberculosis or the enthusiasm of the health workers. Finally, and most important, these will allow you to see how well your patients are managed. Make sure you are one of the enthusiasts who do a good job.

Supplies
Regular and uninterrupted supplies of drugs and materials for microscopy are essential to success.

Training
Repeated central and local training sessions and seminars will compare success rates in diagnosing and treating patients in different places and help health workers to learn from one another.

BCG vaccination
BCG vaccination should be given to all newborn children (with certain exceptions: see page 10) through the national Expanded Programme on Immunization (EPI). All infants should be vaccinated at birth or as early in life as possible.

Family contacts of tuberculosis patients
▶ A patient with a positive sputum smear will often infect members of the family, particularly children. Obviously this is because a family lives in close contact with the patient. If your patient has a positive sputum smear, examine the whole family to find out whether any have been infected. Pay close attention to small children in the family.

▶ On the other hand, if the patient you first diagnose is a child with tuberculosis, examine the whole family to see who may have infected the child. It might be a parent or a grandparent. Of course you will also look for anyone else in the family who has been infected.

▶ Remember that a recently infected child (or adult) may still have a negative tuberculin test and appear well. A positive test, and perhaps illness, may only become apparent later.

▶ Your National Tuberculosis Programme may state a routine for managing family contacts. If so, follow it.

▶ We recommend the guidance and flow charts (Figures 1.4–1.6) that follow. How you manage contacts will depend partly on whether you can do tuberculin tests and whether you can do X-rays.

How to manage family contacts

The flow chart in *Figure 1.4* shows you how to manage a child contact if you can do a tuberculin test.

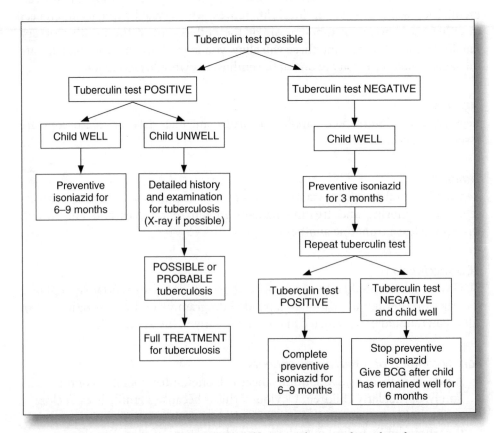

Figure 1.4 *Flow chart for the management of a child contact if you can do a tuberculin test.* (Figure 1.5 shows you how to manage a child contact if you cannot do a tuberculin test.)

Remember the tuberculin test *may be negative* if the child:

▶ has been infected with TB only recently and has not yet become tuberculin positive

▶ is malnourished or ill with another disease

▶ very ill with tuberculosis.

Remember that it is particularly important to give preventive ('prophylactic') isoniazid treatment, as in Figure 1.4, to children aged 5 years or less. These young children are in particular danger from the severe forms of tuberculosis, miliary or meningitis.

The flow chart in *Figure 1.5* shows you how to manage a child contact if you cannot do a tuberculin test.

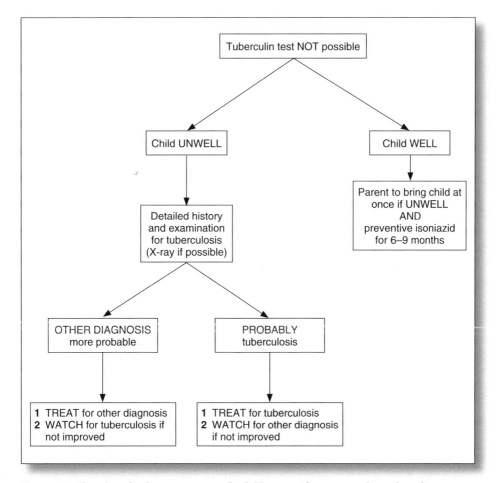

Figure 1.5 *Flow chart for the management of a child contact if you cannot do a tuberculin test.* (Figure 1.4 shows you how to manage a child contact if you can do a tuberculin test.)

The flow chart in *Figure 1.6* shows you how to manage an adult contact. Remember that it is important to examine all adults living in the family home. In particular, remember to examine grandparents, as one of them may be the source of the infection.

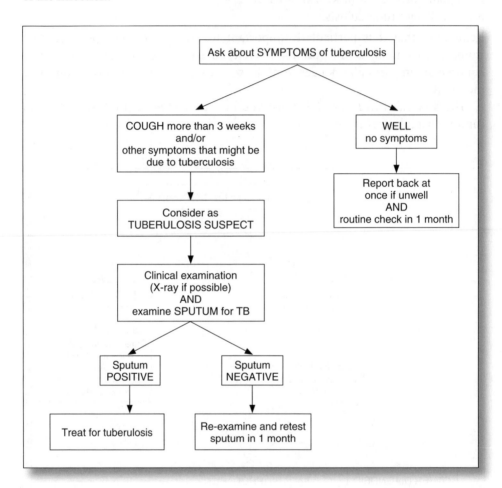

Conclusions

Make sure you are fully familiar with your National Tuberculosis Programme. In particular:

▶ make sure that you test the sputum of any patient who could possibly have tuberculosis
▶ give treatment in accordance with the National Programme. Don't take short cuts or use some new untried chemotherapy. Either may be fatal for your patient.

Coordination of National Tuberculosis Programmes with routine health services

When National Tuberculosis Programmes were started as programmes exclusively devoted to tuberculosis, they rarely managed to cover the whole population. As a result, the WHO recommends that all health programmes in developing countries, including those for tuberculosis, should be carried out through the routine services. Tuberculosis experts will help to plan, supervise, train and retrain. When the programme is fully established, the health care workers in every level of the routine services will be able to identify those who need testing for TB. If the sputum smear is positive, the health care worker will start routine treatment but will refer difficult cases for expert advice.

In any programme, the resources given to tuberculosis must depend on how frequent a health problem it is in that country or area.

Although it is easy to accept this idea in theory, making it really work, or switching over from a previous 'specialized' programme to a programme working well through routine services can be difficult in practice: the aims must be to raise the enthusiasm of health care workers in routine services; to praise their successes; to help them overcome their failures; to train, train and retrain – not only in techniques but, above all, in management; to get workers together regularly to discuss their problems; and above all, to provide leadership to which workers readily respond. All these can help in achieving success. It is best to start by getting diagnosis and treatment working well at selected (pilot) sites and then to expand diagnosis and treatment services progressively to the whole community, including both private and public sectors.

Make sure that you make your own contribution to leadership on developing the programme and making sure it goes on working.

In defeating tuberculosis, management skills are every bit as important as clinical skills. There must be a strong team of experts with the authority and enthusiasm to ensure that the Programme is carried out at all levels of the health service. The team should also be available to give expert advice when needed.

After all, tuberculosis can virtually always be cured, and spread of tuberculosis can be prevented. We have the tools to do the job. This book is to help you to use some of these tools more effectively.

Chapter 2
Tuberculosis in children

When you use this chapter in your work in a health centre or district hospital you will be looking for answers to some or all of the following questions.

1 What happens when a child is first infected with tuberculosis?
2 Is the child I have just seen likely to have tuberculosis?
3 How does tuberculosis present in children?
4 How must I help a child who I think has tuberculosis?

All these questions are linked. To answer one or all of them you need to know how children are infected and the changes that follow a first infection at different ages.

The chapter is therefore set out in five sections, which together will help you to answer the questions you ask yourself:

2.1 Infection with TB (below)
2.2 Identifying the child who might have tuberculosis (page 36)
2.3 Clinical presentation of tuberculosis in children (page 39)
2.4 How you can help and treat children with tuberculosis (page 63)
2.5 HIV infection, AIDS and tuberculosis in children (page 68)

2.1 Infection with TB

How children are infected

From coughing adults

When an adult coughs, many small drops of moisture are forced into the air. If that adult has tuberculosis in the lungs, many of the drops carry bacilli. The largest of the drops fall to the ground. But the smallest, which cannot be seen, remain in the air and move with it.

Outdoors and in well-ventilated rooms, the small drops are carried away in the moving air. But in closed rooms or small spaces they remain in the air, and increase in number as the person continues to cough. Everyone who shares the room with the person who is coughing and breathes the same air runs the risk of breathing in TB. Those nearest to the person coughing are at greatest risk.

The danger is greater when the person coughing does not take any care. Those who cough should cover their mouth and turn away from other people.

A mother with infectious tuberculosis is a danger to her infant or child because she spends a great deal of time close to her infant or child. Nevertheless, both parents may be equally infectious to their children if they share small living or sleeping spaces. The same is true for a teacher in the classroom, a doctor or dentist in the clinic or health centre, a nurse, midwife or health care worker in the home or hospital, a shopkeeper in a shop or a bus driver in a bus, if they have infectious tuberculosis.

When young children are infected, the infection almost always comes from a member of the family group or a near neighbour. When older children are infected and the immediate family is clear, look for a possible source in school, in clinic, in public transport or wherever children come into contact with adults inside buildings or small spaces. In these situations, the bacilli are taken into the lungs with a breath. This is the most frequent pathway to infection. But it is not the only way.

From unboiled cows' milk

TB can reach children in unboiled cows' milk, and infection can then begin in the mouth or intestine. Milk can carry bovine TB if cows in the area have tuberculosis of the udder and the milk is not boiled before use. When the milk is drunk, the primary infection is in the intestine, or sometimes in the tonsils. As mentioned earlier, human infection with bovine bacilli is uncommon in most countries where the prevalence of tuberculosis is high.

Through the skin

This is really very uncommon. Unbroken skin seems to resist TB if they fall upon its surface. But if there has been a recent cut or break, TB may enter and cause an infection as they do in the lungs. As might be expected, skin infection is most likely on exposed surfaces such as the face, legs or feet or, less often, on the arms or hands. It is easy to forget that such a lesion may be tuberculous, even when the nearest lymph nodes are enlarged.

The changes after infection

The primary complex (Figure 2.1a)

When the tiny drops carrying the bacilli are breathed in, they are carried through the air passages to the air sacs (alveoli) of the lungs. There the TB remain and slowly multiply. As that happens, some are carried to the nearest lymph nodes beside the bronchi. In both places, the presence of the bacilli causes a reaction that attracts inflammatory (defence) cells. In about 4–8 weeks there is a small area at the centre of this process where the host tissues are dead (caseation) and around that area is an increasing ring of inflammatory cells, and a tuberculin skin test becomes positive.

The changes in the lung and in the lymph nodes are together known as the primary complex (Figure 2.1a, opposite).

From that time the outcome depends on the ability of the child's immune system to resist the multiplication of the bacilli and limit the amount of caseation. Immunity varies with age, being least in the very young. It also varies with nutrition and HIV infection. Poor nutrition and HIV infection lower body defences.

Most adults and children manage, slowly over many months, to heal both the focus in the lung and that in the lymph nodes. But it takes time and TB can remain inactive but living and capable of multiplication for many years (see Figure 1.3, page 13).

From the time of infection, bacilli escape into the bloodstream and are carried to other parts of the body. Fortunately, disease does not always follow (see below).

We must now look at the changes that occur when the infection progresses and the child becomes ill (diseased).

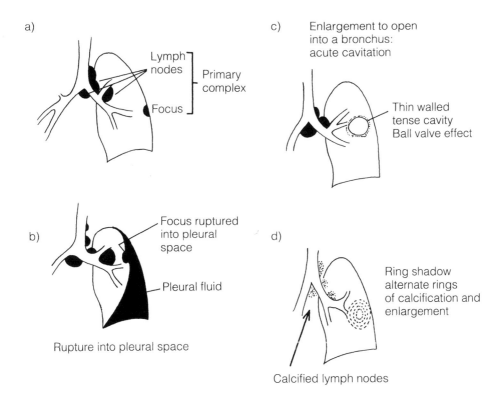

Figure 2.1 *Complications of primary tuberculous complex.* a) Primary lesion in left lung. The lung component is often quite a faint shadow on the X-ray. Note the enlarged hilum and paratracheal lymph nodes. (The drawing is diagrammatic; in an X-ray the shadows are less well defined.) b) Pleural effusion produced by a rupture of the lung component of the primary complex. (In an X-ray the lung lesion is usually hidden by the effusion.) c) Thin-walled cavity resulting from rupture of the primary lung lesion into a bronchus. Bacilli may spread from this cavity to other parts of the lung. d) Rounded coin lesion representing the primary lung component. Later it may become calcified. At this stage, as shown, the hilar and paratracheal lymph nodes may also show calcification. As it calcifies, at some stage there may be rings of calcification around the lung lesion, as shown.

Rupture of a focus into the pleural space (Figure 2.1b)

We have seen that the primary focus forms just below the surface of the lung (pleura). Most do not become larger than 10 mm. Sometimes the focus does get bigger, involving the pleura. The pleura may rupture, allowing caseous material and bacilli to leak into the pleural space.

The result seems to depend on the child's nutrition and degree of tuberculin sensitivity. When nutrition is good and sensitivity is strong, much fluid is produced and a large effusion results. The reaction is much less when sensitivity is low in the young or malnourished child.

The fluid of an effusion is usually absorbed without difficulty. Very occasionally if many bacilli are present the fluid may become purulent and a tuberculous empyema results.

Acute cavitation of focus (Figure 2.1c)

When immunity is poor, as in young, HIV-infected or malnourished children, the primary focus may increase in size. Instead of leaking into the pleural space, it may open into a small bronchus and the caseous material is discharged by coughing.

During this process there may be a stage when air can enter the small cavity when the patient is breathing in but cannot escape when he or she is breathing out. This results in the formation of a small thin-walled cavity.

This process can spread TB to other parts of the lungs. Spread may also occur by the erosion of the tuberculous nodes through the bronchial wall. Caseous material and TB from the nodes then spread through the bronchi to other parts of the lungs.

Very rarely, a child can suffocate from caseous material that suddenly blocks both main bronchi. Emergency bronchoscopy, if available, could save such a child. If this is not available, turn the child upside down and percuss the chest with the open hand to try to help the child to cough up the material and clear the bronchi.

Progressive lung disease is particularly likely in young children and those who are HIV-infected or malnourished. It may proceed so rapidly that the child dies from tuberculous pneumonia before developing signs of blood-spread disease such as disseminated tuberculosis or tuberculous meningitis.

Ring or coin shadow (Figure 2.1d)

Very occasionally in older children (and found only by X-ray examination), a round coin-like lesion can be seen in the lung field. Sometimes the edge is calcified, or a series of zones of calcification may be seen, representing periods of healing and extension. This can remain unchanged for long periods. The lesion may then completely or partially calcify.

The lymph nodes at the root of the lung (Figure 2.2)

Bacilli from the primary focus reach the lymph nodes by direct drainage. These nodes lie near to the air passages (bronchi). Both the nodes and the air passages get larger towards the centre (hilum) of the lung.

The bacilli in the nodes cause a change which is similar to that in the focus in the lung, and the node becomes larger and may soften.

In very young children the nodes can press upon and narrow the soft air passage, resulting in airway obstruction which presents as loud wheezing. In some children the narrowing can be so severe that it causes collapse of that part of the lung *(Figures 2.2* and *2.3).*

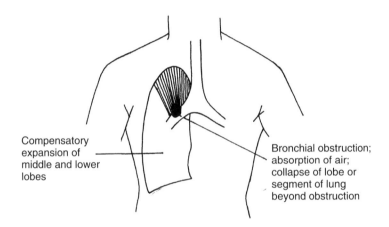

Compensatory expansion of middle and lower lobes

Bronchial obstruction; absorption of air; collapse of lobe or segment of lung beyond obstruction

Figure 2.2 *Complications of the mediastinal lymph nodes of the primary complex: collapse of right upper lobe with expansion of middle and lower lobes to compensate.*

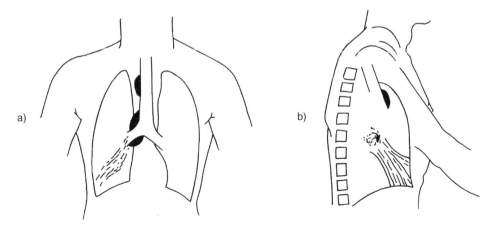

a)

b)

Figure 2.3 *Complications of the mediastinal lymph nodes of the primary complex: collapse of the middle lobe of the right lung.* The nature of the shadow is much clearer in a lateral X-ray film (b).

In the older child, a node can break through the wall of the bronchus. When that happens, the soft contents of the node can leak into the air passage and the material containing bacilli can be drawn further into the lung as the child breathes in. So the disease is spread to other parts of the lung, leading to a bronchopneumonic picture *(Figure 2.4)*. This method of spread is common in young, poorly nourished children.

If the child's defences are better, there is merely an extensive exudate (outpouring) of fluid and cells into that part of the lung. This is due to hypersensitivity to the TB or to tuberculoprotein in the caseous material. These exudates, as seen on the X-ray, later clear completely *(Figure 2.5)*.

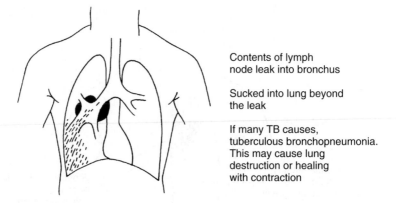

Contents of lymph node leak into bronchus

Sucked into lung beyond the leak

If many TB causes, tuberculous bronchopneumonia. This may cause lung destruction or healing with contraction

Figure 2.4 *Complications of the mediastinal lymph nodes of the primary complex: erosion (bursting) of the mediastinal lymph nodes into a bronchus.* The material has been sucked into a bronchus beyond the leak. This has led to tuberculous bronchopneumonia.

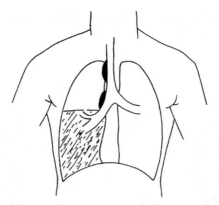

Figure 2.5 *Complications of tuberculous lymph nodes of the primary complex: erosion of tuberculous lymph nodes into a bronchus and inhalation of contents.* This has caused an extensive exudate (outpouring of fluid) into the right lower lobe. The child may be much less ill than would be suggested from the X-ray. The shadow may clear slowly but completely over a number of months. On the X-ray alone you cannot distinguish this shadow from a very extensive tuberculous pneumonia, but a child with tuberculous pneumonia would be much more ill. Both are different from an acute bacterial pneumonia, which comes on quickly and improves with antibiotics. The large hilar and paratracheal nodes on the X-ray make tuberculosis much more probable.

Occasionally the contents of the lymph nodes are firmer and simply stick into the bronchus so that air can pass the narrowed space when the child breathes in, but the gap is closed and the air is trapped when the child breathes out ('obstructive hyperinflation') *(Figure 2.6)*. This blows up the lung beyond the narrowing, although in most cases this does not last long. However, the block may become complete, in which case the lung collapses, or the lesion clears up.

Any of these forms of pneumonia, exudates or collapse may result in damage to the bronchi of that lobe or segment, which may give rise to bronchiectasis *(Figure 2.7)*.

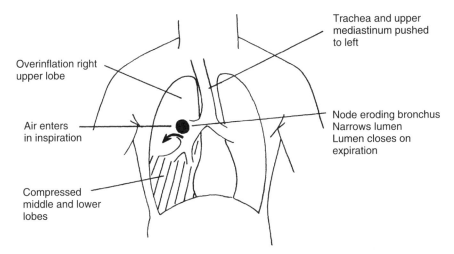

Figure 2.6 *Complications of tuberculous lymph nodes of the primary complex: ball-valve obstruction of the upper lobe bronchus by an enlarged hilar lymph node.* This allows air into, but not out of, the right upper lobe. The right upper lobe is blown up (distended) by 'obstructive emphysema'. Note the compressed middle and lower lobes, and that the trachea is pushed to the opposite side. On the X-ray, the inflated area looks blacker than the rest of the lung and has few lung markings.

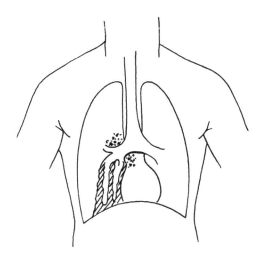

Figure 2.7 *Complications of tuberculous lymph nodes of the primary complex: bronchiectasis in a collapsed right lower lobe due to an old tuberculous primary complex.* Calcification of hilar lymph nodes (showing more intensely white on the X-ray) suggests the cause of the collapse. Because the lower lobe bronchus is poorly drained by gravity, there is often secondary infection and symptoms of bronchiectasis. The same may occur in the middle lobe.

29

Other complications of lymph node disease (Figure 2.8)

So far the complications we have described have resulted from damage of the bronchi by the lymph nodes. But two other structures in the chest may be affected. There is a group of large lymph nodes in the space where the main windpipe (trachea) divides to supply a branch to each lung. At the front this group is in close contact with the back of the pericardium which surrounds the heart. At the back they are near the oesophagus as it goes down to pass through the diaphragm to the stomach. If this group of nodes enlarges and softens with tuberculosis, it may involve the pericardium. The node contents may leak into the pericardium, producing a pericardial effusion *(Figure 2.8)*. Very occasionally, instead of reaching to the front, the mass of nodes becomes attached to the oesophagus, resulting in a pouch.

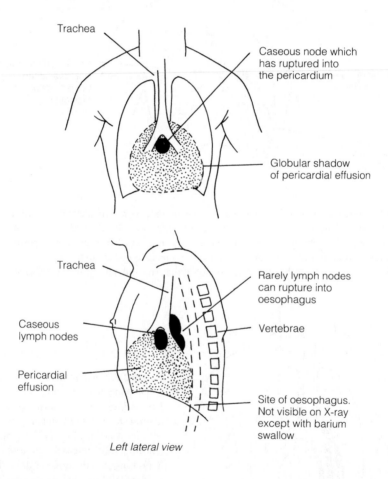

Figure 2.8 *Complications of tuberculous lymph nodes of the primary complex: pericardial effusion due to rupture of a tuberculous lymph node into the pericardium.* We show the lymph node in the diagram but you would not see it in the X-ray.

Blood spread of bacilli (Figure 2.9)

During the time the primary complex is forming and for some time afterwards, bacilli escape into the bloodstream from both the focus and the nodes. This may occur either by eroding a blood vessel in the lesion or through the lymphatics.

The bloodstream carries the TB to distant parts of the body such as the liver, spleen, bones, brain and kidneys. This process ceases as the primary focus and its nodes heal, but it can continue for many months. Most of these bacilli remain dormant in small tubercles and do not cause any clinical illness and are healed by the child's own defensive powers.

Very young children have weak defences, which may be further reduced by malnutrition or by other infectious diseases, particularly HIV infection, measles or whooping cough. In these children primary infection may be rapidly followed by disseminated tuberculosis and/or tuberculous meningitis. These are rapidly fatal diseases if not properly treated. If the child's defences are better, or fewer bacilli spread, one of the more chronic lesions may present after months or years. The more chronic lesions may present months or years later. These include tuberculosis of bones, joints, kidneys or a variety of other organs.

Any of these forms, including disseminated tuberculosis or meningitis, may occur at any time in life if there is a dormant (sleeping) lesion somewhere in the body and the patient's resistance is lowered.

Tuberculosis of the cervical lymph nodes is more common in Africa and Asia but occurs in all locations. The bacilli are most likely to have arrived at the lymph nodes through either the lymphatics or the blood.

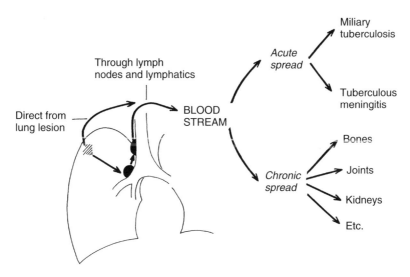

Figure 2.9 *Blood spread of TB.* This can occur either a) directly to the bloodstream from the lung lesion or b) from the lung lesion through the lymphatics to the lymph nodes, and then from the nodes through the lymphatics, which eventually empty into the bloodstream. Acute spread of many TB may rapidly result in fatal miliary tuberculosis or tuberculous meningitis. Chronic spread of fewer TB may cause disease in bones, joints, kidneys, etc. months or years later.

Some stories about primary tuberculosis and its complications

A family outbreak of tuberculosis

A family of a father, mother, two boys, aged 7 and 3, and a baby girl of 9 months, lived in a provincial town. The 3-year-old boy, Ong, became unwell. He had a low fever. Sometimes he ate a meal normally, sometimes he refused all food. His mother took him to a local doctor. The doctor found nothing definite, but gave him penicillin.

After 7–10 days, Ong began to vomit. The doctor sent him to the District Hospital, where he was admitted. On examination he was fretful, thin and dehydrated. There were no other abnormal physical signs. X-ray of the chest showed enlargement of shadows at the left lung root. Lumbar puncture showed 186 cells per mm^3 and 100 mg protein%. (Culture later grew TB.) This, with the X-ray, strongly suggested tuberculous meningitis. Treatment was started immediately and the child made a complete recovery. When the diagnosis was made, the family was examined. The father's sputum was negative but the mother's sputum smear was positive and her chest X-ray showed extensive tuberculosis.

The brother, Sak, aged 7, was found to be unwell and listless and he had a slight cough. Chest X-ray showed a primary complex on the right side. He rapidly improved with treatment.

The baby girl, Shinta, was well. She was given isoniazid (5 mg/kg/day) for 6 months to prevent disease.

All the family took their treatment regularly. The mother's sputum was negative at 2 and 5 months after starting treatment, indicating cure. The children's symptoms cleared and they gained weight, showing a good clinical response to treatment.

Comment: This family was very well managed. When the first child's illness did not improve with penicillin, the doctor referred him to hospital. The hospital doctor realized that the child was ill and admitted him. The doctor thought of the possibility of tuberculosis. This suspicion was increased after the chest X-ray. The lumbar puncture showed that there was early meningitis. The doctor then went on to examine the family, which revealed two more cases, who were then cured. Disease was prevented in the youngest member of the family by giving preventive chemotherapy.

Primary tuberculosis with bronchial erosion

A girl, Sandra, aged 4 years, was an only child. Her mother took her to hospital because she was losing weight and had had a cough for about 2 months. On examination the child looked thin. There was a suspicion that the left side of the chest did not move as well as the right: the air

cont'd ▶

entry on that side was reduced. The child could not produce any sputum. X-ray showed scattered areas of patchy shadowing throughout the left lung and some enlargement of the root of the lung. The doctor started Sandra on anti-tuberculosis chemotherapy. Her general health improved rapidly and she recovered completely, with no evidence of lung damage.

The mother and father were examined but had no evidence of tuberculosis. Sandra often visited a grandmother. The mother confirmed that the grandmother had a chronic cough. The grandmother was brought to the hospital and was found to have tuberculosis, as her sputum was positive for TB. In due course she was cured by treatment.

Comment: A story of 2 months' cough and loss of weight made pneumonia an unlikely diagnosis. Tuberculosis was more probable. This combined with the X-ray findings made this diagnosis certain.

Collapsed right, middle and lower lobes due to caseous material from a tuberculous lymph node obstructing the bronchi

A girl, Bimla, aged 12, began to feel ill while at school. She felt feverish and had a headache. She also developed a dry cough. A doctor saw her and gave her penicillin. She improved slightly for a few days, but then the cough and headache came back. The doctor sent her to the District Hospital, where she was admitted.

On examination, Bimla had a fever of 38.9°C. There was decreased movement of the right side of the chest. The heart and trachea were displaced to that side and the breath sounds were greatly decreased. This suggested collapse of one or more lobes. Chest X-ray showed collapse of the right, middle and lower lobes.

The hospital doctor at first gave Bimla penicillin.

There were no facilities for bronchoscopy at the hospital. Something was obstructing Bimla's right lower lobe and middle lobe bronchi, which might have been caseous material coming from tuberculous lymph nodes. A fit of coughing resulting in Bimla coughing up some 'cheesy' material. The doctor sent this for microscopy and TB were identified.

The doctor therefore changed the treatment to anti-tuberculosis chemotherapy. The child's fever began to come down at once.

After the fit of coughing Bimla's right chest moved better and both sides now seemed normal. Repeat X-ray showed that the lobes had re-expanded. Bimla's temperature became normal in 10 days. She completed full treatment and remained well.

Her family were examined but no-one else was found to have tuberculosis.

The time course and risks of primary infection

We know something about the usual time course of tuberculosis by following a group of European children whose time of infection was known, for a long period of time after their infection. The common timetable of the complications of primary tuberculosis is set out in *Figure 2.10*. This diagram also gives some indication of the factors that increased the risk of the most serious complications. These risks were found in children in a well-nourished population before effective treatment was available. Risks are greater in any population where malnutrition or HIV infection is common. Figure 2.10 shows the time relationships of the development of the primary complex after the child has been infected, and that most go on to heal. However, complications can arise from the focus in the lung, from the lymph nodes and then spread to other organs, brain, bone and, much later, the kidneys. The figure also give an indication of how long after infection complications are most likely to occur, and of the things that make a primary infection more dangerous by reducing the body's power to resist the multiplication of the TB.

At present it is uncertain how far the timetable given in Figure 2.10 applies to children in developing countries, but it nevertheless provides a useful framework.

The effect of age at infection, nutrition and other infections and infestations

The power to resist infection depends on the ability of the child's immune system to overcome an invading organism. The child's immunity depends on their age, nutrition and the presence of other infections (especially HIV infection) or infestations. Disease can develop rapidly in children with poor immunity, whereas in other children the clinical presentation is that of a chronic disease.

In tuberculosis the bacilli grow slowly over weeks and months rather than days. So the effects and signs of the disease appear slowly.

The changes that follow the first infection are described above. We also showed how most of those who have a first infection with tuberculosis manage to heal it. Their bodies have indeed learned to respond more quickly to future attacks by TB. If they should get another infection, the body's quicker defence prevents the spread of bacilli to other organs, as occurs during the first infection. This is probably the reason why BCG vaccination, which produces a harmless form of primary infection, reduces the frequency of disseminated tuberculosis and tuberculous meningitis.

But the defences do not work so well at every age. They are relatively poor at birth, improving slowly for the first 5 years or so of life. Up to 5 years of age the child is less able at preventing blood spread, though this gradually improves with age. A well-nourished child seems good at preventing the spread of disease within the lung itself. After puberty the body is better at preventing blood spread, but is more inclined to develop pulmonary TB with cavities. Poorly nourished children may develop severe cavitating lung disease at an early age.

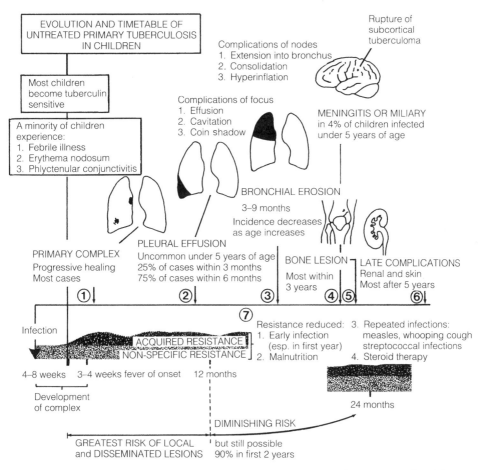

Figure 2.10 *Evolution and timetable of untreated primary tuberculous infection.* (Reproduced from Miller, FJW. *Tuberculosis in Children*, Churchill Livingstone, 1983.) Note that this time course is based on observations on European children. It is not yet clear how far this time course applies in other settings but it nevertheless provides a useful framework.

Throughout life the body only responds to infection in the best way if it is well nourished with an adequate supply of proper food. At any age, insufficient food, leading to malnutrition, reduces the power of the body to respond to its full capacity. This increases not only the seriousness of disease but also the chance that the patient will die of the disease. Severe worm infestation, particularly with intestinal parasites, can be a cause of malnutrition, particularly if the amount of food eaten is only just enough.

HIV infection is the most important factor that reduces a child's immunity and increases the chances of tuberculosis. If other infections, especially measles and whooping cough, occur while the child has a primary infection, that disease may extend and disseminated tuberculosis or meningitis develops.

2.2 Identifying the child who might have tuberculosis

When to think of tuberculosis (see other sections for more detail)

It is not enough to understand how children are infected with tuberculosis or how the disease may spread. You must know when to think that a child who comes to see you may have tuberculosis. Remember to think of it whenever you see a child who is thin or has:

▶ a chronic cough that has been present for 3 weeks or longer or is getting worse
▶ failed to gain weight or has lost weight for more than 4 weeks (a weight chart is valuable)
▶ lost energy and possibly some weight over 2–3 months
▶ has had a fever or raised temperature for more than a week without any explanation
▶ any or all of the first three signs and physical signs of chest disease – wheezing, decreased air movement or dullness on one side of the chest
▶ a swollen abdomen, especially if a lump is felt and if the lump remains after treatment for worms
▶ chronic diarrhoea with large pale stools, which has not responded to treatment for worms or giardiasis
▶ a limp on walking; a stiff spine and is unwilling to bend his or her back
▶ spinal hump with or without stiffness in walking
▶ swelling of knee, ankle, wrist, elbow, shoulder, rib or any bone or joint not due to injury
▶ a swollen, painless, firm or soft lymph node swelling, sometimes with smaller lymph nodes near to it and sometimes matted to it
▶ a lymph node abscess which may be affecting or coming through the skin
▶ one or more soft swellings under the skin; these are not painful; the skin may have broken, leaving an ulcer with sharply cut edges and usually a clean base
▶ a discharging sinus (wound) near any joint
▶ headache and irritability, occasional vomiting, child wishes to be left alone and gradually becomes less rousable over 2–3 weeks
▶ slow onset of weakness in one arm or leg or side of face.

Important points to remember

▶ Tuberculosis and malnutrition go together: tuberculosis can cause kwashiorkor, xerophthalmia or vitamin B deficiency.
▶ The slow onset of typhoid (enteric) fever or paratyphoid can have the same appearance as tuberculosis.
▶ Tuberculosis may present as a chronic or repeated lung infections.
▶ Malaria and tuberculosis may be present together in the same child or one may be mistaken for the other.
▶ Swellings of lymph nodes such as lymphoma can resemble tuberculosis.

▶ Your patient may have more than one infection or infestation, and different parasites are found in different regions – be aware of the types in your locality.

▶ It is essential to consider whether a child may have tuberculosis complicating HIV infection. In children, HIV-related lung diseases may closely resemble tuberculosis.

How to plan action – recording of a child suspected to have tuberculosis

Always be ready to suspect tuberculosis. Record the information, history and the physical examination systematically as follows. (Preferably use any standard tuberculosis records for children produced by your National Tuberculosis Programme.

▶ Names of patient, father and mother
▶ Address or location of house
▶ Age and sex of patient
▶ Weight and height – is the weight within the ideal range for the child's age (according to the 'Road to Health' chart)?
▶ BCG, history of injection, presence of scar
▶ Family history of tuberculosis, or suggestive of tuberculosis; remember to ask whether any grandparents have a chronic cough, and about relatives who have died recently and may have had a cough
▶ Duration of present illness
▶ Parents' complaint concerning child: cough, sweat, loss of weight, appetite or energy, limp, change in behaviour or temper, headache, lumps or swellings
▶ Child's symptoms and signs found on examination:
  – abdomen: pain, swelling, enlargement of spleen or liver
  – chest: cough, wheeze or pain; any dullness to percussion suggesting consolidation or fluid
  – limbs: swelling of joints, pain on walking, stiffness
  – spine: stiffness or hump
  – skin: ulcers or sores; swollen lymph nodes in neck, groin or armpit
▶ X-ray. Whenever possible obtain an X-ray of the chest. You must consider the results in relation to all the other clinical evidence. Interpretation of children's X-rays can be difficult. We give some guidance in the notes on Figures 2.1 to 2.8 (pages 25–30). When X-ray is not possible, you may have to decide on the basis of clinical evidence alone.
▶ Children do not usually produce sputum. If they are able to do so, however, it should be sent for microscopic examination. The same applies to any other fluid obtainable. If you cannot do it on the spot, you can send suitable specimens to the nearest large hospital or laboratory. This will depend on your local organization.

▶ When facilities are available for TB culture, it is recommended that gastric aspiration is performed on all young children suspected of having tuberculosis, if sputum cannot be obtained otherwise. (For details see Appendix F.) This investigation may be distressing for the child.

▶ When you suspect tuberculosis, if you can, send the child to a centre where full investigation is possible. However, we realize this may not be possible in many places, in which case you will find guidance below.

▶ It is extremely important to do everything possible to avoid the spread of HIV; in particular, never re-use needles or syringes.

In areas where HIV and malnutrition are common, the primary infection in the lung and lymph nodes often goes on to progressive disease. Under these circumstances more children will present with chest complaints and loss of weight. But tuberculosis does not always cause dramatic physical signs in the lungs.

Cough is usually present. Wheeze (due to lymph node pressure on the bronchi) is gentle and is heard when breathing both in and out. Children very rarely spit blood. (When they do it may be due to whooping cough.) The child's temperature may be raised, but very high fevers are not common. If you suspect trouble in the chest and the child cannot be moved to a larger hospital, then you have to do the best you can. If you can, obtain an X-ray. When you see the film you must judge it together with all the other information about the child. This includes the family history (known tuberculosis or possible tuberculosis), the length of the history of the illness, the appearance of the child, the physical signs and the results of the tuberculin test (if available).

The following make it more likely that you are *not* dealing with tuberculosis but with another bacterial infection: a) short history of illness, b) rapid breathing and chest wall indrawing, c) acutely ill child and d) no history suggestive of possible tuberculosis in family or neighbours.

The following make it *more* likely that you are dealing with tuberculosis: a) illness of some weeks duration, b) child chronically, rather than acutely, ill, c) few physical signs, d) a family history of known or possible tuberculosis and e) a strongly positive tuberculin test. Look also for signs of tuberculosis in other parts of the body.

Scoring systems

Various scoring systems have been developed to help in the diagnosis of tuberculosis in a child. Although these systems have been widely used, their accuracy has not been validated. Furthermore, many of them rely on the contribution of the tuberculin skin test to the score, a test that is rarely available in reality. In areas where there is a high prevalence of HIV infection these scoring systems perform particularly poorly, resulting in the over-diagnosis of tuberculosis and incorrect treatment of many children. For this reason, we do not recommend using these scoring systems; rather the emphasis is on taking a careful history, examining the child, and taking a chest X-ray. By carefully using these elements, the diagnosis of tuberculosis can be easily made in the majority of children.

> **Important note**
>
> This plan of treatment will only succeed if you observe the patient closely. Record all changes in his or her behaviour, temperature, weight, symptoms and signs of disease.

2.3 Clinical presentation of tuberculosis in children

Above we have given an overall impression of the child with tuberculosis. In this section we go into more detail. We review some of the many ways in which tuberculosis may present clinically in the child.

In the lungs

As in adults, tuberculosis in children affects the lungs more frequently than any other part of the body. This is because the usual route of infection is by breathing in air that contains bacilli and the extension of the primary complex that follows the infection.

In spite of this, when the child is examined there are frequently no physical signs or symptoms that indicate with certainty that the child has tuberculosis. The only complete proof that the child has tuberculosis is finding the TB, which is particularly challenging in children.

In the health centre or small hospital the diagnosis must often be made on clinical grounds alone. So in these conditions the history and clinical examination become all important. It is well worth taking time and trouble over the history, which is often the most important clue to the diagnosis. Listen carefully to what the mother says. If there are signs or symptoms of illness this usually indicates that the tuberculosis is extending. The extension may be in the focus in the lung, in the lymph nodes into which the focus drains, or in the body generally.

When first seen, the complaint is frequently that the child has a cough which has been present for 3 weeks or longer and is not improving. This is frequently accompanied by loss of weight or failure to gain weight, or the child has lost their normal level of energy and activity. They may sweat and have a fever. The cough is usually non-productive, such that sputum is hard to obtain for examination. Children with tuberculosis practically never cough up blood or blood-stained sputum. All this has usually been present for some weeks before the child is brought to be seen.

There may be signs of vitamin deficiency, which may have appeared either before or after the general change in health was noticed.

The family history is important. Do the parents or grandparents have any history of cough or have they had any treatment for tuberculosis? Are any neighbours known to have a chronic cough or tuberculosis? Sometimes a family history of tuberculosis may be suppressed. Have there been any recent deaths in the family?

When you examine the child you must adapt your approach to the age of the child. Young children are best examined while being held by the parent; older children may sit or lie on a bed.

Always remember that you may learn far more by carefully watching than by any other way. Train yourself to watch the child's behaviour, their physique (height and weight by age), skin, hair and breathing rate.

▶ Is there a wheeze or a cough and if so is the cough loud or soft?
▶ Does the chest move equally on both sides?
▶ Does the child seem to have any pain on breathing or elsewhere?
▶ If you tap (percuss) the chest with your finger, can you feel any difference on one side or the other – is there dullness which may show that there is fluid or solid lung in that area?
▶ If you listen with a stethoscope, can you detect if more air is entering one side of the chest than the other, or can you hear a wheeze as when there is narrowing of the air passages?
▶ Sometimes you will hear moist or wet sounds if there is fluid in the air passage.

You must remember that whatever physical signs you find, these only help you to understand what is happening in one or both lungs in a mechanical sense. The signs do not tell you the cause of the changes.

All the information that you have now collected must be carefully considered and the clinical diagnosis of tuberculosis suspected. This will then guide your next action. Is it necessary to do a tuberculin skin test or a chest X-ray? Should the child be referred to a hospital for more investigations?

Disseminated tuberculosis

Disseminated tuberculosis is the result of heavy spread of bacilli via the blood stream, which then seed into the lungs, liver, spleen and brain. The earliest symptoms of disseminated tuberculosis are loss of energy and activity, weight loss and fever. On examination there may be an enlarged liver or spleen, and even signs of meningitis. There may not be any signs in the chest until the disease is far advanced. The X-ray of the chest, if this is possible, may show millet-sized shadows dotted throughout both lungs (called miliary tuberculosis), although this may not be obvious in the early stages. A few cases may have signs of tuberculosis in the other organs but nothing clearly wrong on the chest X-ray. Lymphocytic interstitial pneumonia in an HIV-infected child can give a very similar clinical and radiological picture and should be kept in mind.

Three stories about disseminated tuberculosis

Jumbe

A 6-month-old boy, Jumbe, was brought to hospital by his mother, who said that he had had a cough for a month or more and was losing weight. He vomited occasionally. Two weeks previously the baby's right ear began to discharge. About the same time the mother noticed lumps on both sides of his neck. They did not seem painful.

The doctor asked about the family. The mother then said that the father had been admitted to hospital with pulmonary tuberculosis 3 months earlier. The boy had not been given BCG or preventive therapy with isoniazid after the diagnosis of his father's tuberculosis. He had not seen his father since.

On examination the baby was alert but had obviously lost weight. The external meatus of the right ear was filled with granulation tissue. The skin was ulcerated. There were several enlarged lymph nodes on each side of the neck. The anterior fontanel felt full. The doctor found nothing abnormal in the lungs. The liver was enlarged two finger-breadths below the costal margin. With his history, the doctor thought tuberculosis was likely. X-ray of the chest showed miliary tuberculosis.

Lumbar puncture showed 9 lymphocytes per mm^3 and 65 mg of protein% in the cerebrospinal fluid. TB were seen in the cerebrospinal fluid and in the discharge from the ear.

Treatment was begun at once. For the next week Jumbe was difficult to feed. He vomited occasionally. His abdomen became rather distended and the doctor could feel a mass across the upper abdomen. But then, with continuing treatment, Jumbe gradually improved. By the 4th month the mass could no longer be felt. The neck nodes remained small and firm. He made a complete recovery except that he was left with a perforated eardrum. X-ray at a year showed extensive calcification in the abdomen and the neck but the chest was normal, with no calcification.

Comment: The father had obviously infected Jumbe. At the time of the father's diagnosis, Jumbe should have received isoniazid (5 mg/kg/day) for up to 9 months for optimum effect, to prevent him developing the disease. Being 3 months of age he was at particularly high risk for developing disseminated tuberculosis and meningitis. By getting the family history the hospital doctor immediately made the right diagnosis and treated the abdominal, ear, miliary and early tuberculous meningitis successfully.

Koresi

Koresi was 2 years old when his mother first brought him to hospital. He was an only son. His mother's first child had died of whooping cough at 5 months of age. Koresi had been watched at a clinic in his village from birth. He had gained weight well in his first 6 months but then more slowly. In his second year he was away from his own village. At about 18 months of age he started to lose weight slowly. He had attacks of fever, cough and diarrhoea. Finally, just at the end of his second year, his mother brought him to hospital.

His X-ray showed widespread miliary tuberculosis. He responded well to treatment. The source of infection was not found.

Koresi had been followed from birth. His weight chart *(Figure 2.11)* shows the loss of weight in the months before diagnosis and the rapid gain after treatment was started.

Imam

Imam, a twin boy aged 4, had been vaguely unwell since an attack of measles 8 months earlier. Then one day his mother found a painless swelling above the inner end of his right clavicle. She had also noticed that he had had several crops of tiny painless non-irritable spots on his face, body and limbs. The swelling in his neck then became soft and discharged some creamy pus. He was sent to hospital.

On examination, Imam's general condition appeared good and his temperature was normal. A swelling with a central softening was found in the right side of the neck above the clavicle, and a small firm node was found on the left side. There were many small rather scaly spots scattered over his body and limbs. They seemed to be in the skin and were 1–3 mm in diameter. X-ray of his chest showed a partly calcified lesion in the right upper lobe, enlarged right paratracheal lymph nodes with early calcification, and miliary tuberculosis. There was also calcification in the soft tissue swelling above his right clavicle. Pus was obtained from the abscess above the clavicle. Many TB were seen on microscopic examination.

On treatment, the wound healed and both the skin lesions and the miliary lesions of the lungs disappeared. Imam made an uninterrupted recovery.

The family were examined. Both parents were healthy. His twin brother and elder sister were healthy. The source of his infection was unknown.

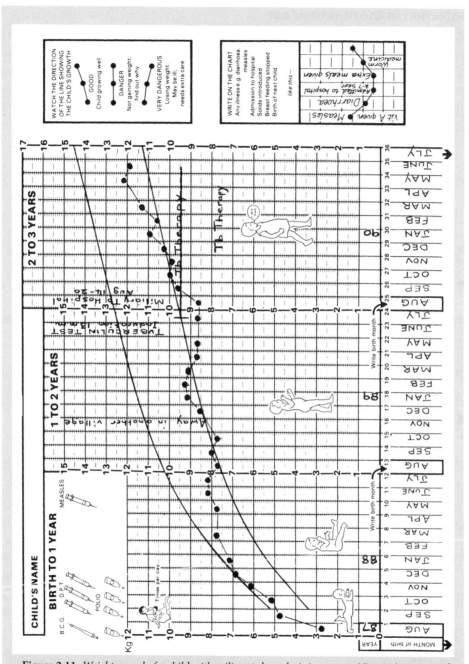

Figure 2.11 *Weight record of a child with miliary tuberculosis in western Nigeria* (courtesy of Professor David Morley).

Infection in the mouth or ear

Although most children have their primary infection in the lungs and come to the health service with signs of chest disease, some get tuberculosis in other parts of the body. Also remember that the primary infection can occur anywhere on the skin or on any mucous membrane where bacilli can lodge. When that happens, the first sign is nearly always painless swelling, and sometimes softening, of the lymph nodes draining the primary focus. If, for example, the focus is in the mouth or on a tonsil, the nodes in the neck that drain the area become enlarged.

The ear and mastoid process can become infected in three ways.

▶ Bacilli may be swept up the Eustachian tube when an infant or young child is feeding. The focus may then be inside the ear and the node is between the mastoid process and the angle of the jaw. The ear runs. The facial nerve may be involved so that the face on that side seems flat.

▶ If that happens in a child who has already had a primary infection in some other site, there is still a chronic discharge from the ear but no enlarged node.

▶ Tuberculosis may affect the mastoid by blood spread from a primary focus in the chest.

Suspect tuberculosis in any child with a chronic painless discharge from the ear. Take an ear swab and have it examined for TB.

Abdominal tuberculosis

Abdominal tuberculosis in children can begin in different ways:

▶ through blood spread to the abdomen from a primary focus in the lung
▶ from the milk of tuberculous cows that has been given to the child without first being boil.

Children very rarely get intestinal ulceration complicating primary disease.

The primary lesion may be in the intestine and the nodes in the mesentery. The nodes enlarge, can soften and may leak their tuberculous contents into the abdominal cavity. The result is free fluid (ascites) and a swollen abdomen. In other cases, the nodes, instead of rupturing, cause the loops of bowel to stick together. This can cause pain and attacks of bowel obstruction, which may eventually become complete. As the intestines become stuck to each other they may form masses which can be felt through the abdominal wall.

You must distinguish swelling of the abdomen due to tuberculosis from other causes such as stretching of weak muscles in malnutrition or intestinal infestation.

A boy with abdominal tuberculosis

Wong, aged 9, was brought to hospital by his parents. He had been vaguely unwell for about 6 months. He had a poor appetite and occasional attacks of right-sided abdominal pain. For the past few days his symptoms had increased. His doctor had found his temperature to be 39°C.   *cont'd* ▶

Wong's parents were healthy, but an aunt had been found to have pulmonary tuberculosis 4 months earlier.

On examination, Wong's abdomen was distended and was rather tender on the right side. Liver and spleen could not be felt. X-ray of chest and abdomen was normal. No occult blood was found in the faeces.

His condition remained unchanged for 3 days and he continued to run a fever. By the third day there was evidence of free fluid in the abdomen.

On the fourth day an aspirate was taken of the free abdominal fluid (ascites) which was examined and found to be suggestive of tuberculosis. By the fifth day the doctor decided to treat the illness as abdominal tuberculosis. Within 48 hours of starting treatment Wong began to improve. His temperature began to fall, he began to eat, and his abdominal swelling decreased. After this he made a steady recovery. He completed treatment and remained well.

Tuberculosis of the lymph nodes

How tuberculosis of lymph nodes arises

This is a relatively frequent site of disease, after pulmonary disease. Most often the disease affects the nodes in the neck but sometimes it affects the nodes in the armpits or groin. When this happens, there is likely to be a primary focus in the area that drains into the swollen nodes. You should look carefully for it. In other cases, the cervical nodes above the clavicle are involved through spread by the lymphatics from the mediastinal nodes in the chest or through the bloodstream; in this case, the primary focus is in the lung. Tuberculosis can cause generalized lymph node enlargement in an HIV-infected child.

How tuberculosis of lymph nodes presents in the child

Localized enlargement of lymph nodes

Enlargement of the nodes is usually slow and painless. Children may be seen with two forms of presentation, depending on the state of the nodes.

▶ The first group comes soon after the nodes have been found to be enlarged. There is one large node and several smaller ones near to it. The skin is not involved and the node feels firm.

▶ The second group comes later when the nodes are matted together and the skin is fixed over them. These nodes are then becoming soft to form abscesses which will come through the skin and burst if they are not opened and the pus removed. The abscess is a 'cold' abscess – it is not hot or tender, but fluctuant (showing that it contains liquid). Draining the abscess through a small incision will preserve the skin and result in a smaller scar as healing occurs with anti-tuberculosis treatment.

Generalized enlargement of the lymph nodes

Before the appearance of HIV, generalized lymph node enlargement was only very rarely due to tuberculosis. In HIV infection, the child has reduced immunity and a primary infection with tuberculosis may spread and cause generalized lymph node enlargement.

However, remember that general enlargement is often the first sign of HIV infection itself, even without tuberculosis. If in doubt, examine the mother, who may show clinical evidence of AIDS.

Distinguishing lymph node enlargement from other conditions

Nodes become infected for many reasons and tuberculosis must be distinguished from:

▶ acute septic inflammation, in which the child is more acutely ill and the node swelling is rapid, painful and tender to touch; there is usually some septic lesion in the area drained by the node (perhaps hidden in the hair)

▶ the firm smooth swelling of Burkitt's lymphoma arises from the upper or lower jaw; it occurs in children in tropical Africa

▶ the swelling of leukaemia, which is usually generalized and with signs of bruising and anaemia

▶ in lymphoma the first nodes affected are usually just above the collar bone or in the armpit; they are painless and feel very hard, and the liver and spleen are also often enlarged.

Remember that the axillary (armpit) lymph nodes on the same side often enlarge after BCG vaccination. Ask the mother and look for the BCG scar.

You will often have to make the diagnosis purely on clinical grounds but this is usually not difficult. A fine-needle aspiration is useful in making the definitive diagnosis. Insert a needle with a syringe attached into the node and try to suck out material. Even if you get no material, use the needle to make a smear on a slide. The smear is fixed and stained. This is used to make the correct diagnosis, including tuberculosis. Culture the aspirate if possible. If the diagnosis is still uncertain, take a biopsy from the node.

Tuberculosis of the brain and spinal cord

Tuberculosis begins in the central nervous system when TB spreads through the bloodstream, reaches nervous tissue and local reaction forms a tuberculoma. This may cause symptoms because of its size, like a malignant tumour, or it may burst into the space surrounding the brain or spinal cord and cause meningitis. The younger the child, the greater the risk and the more difficult the diagnosis.

Tuberculous meningitis

When a tuberculoma in the brain leaks or ruptures, living or dead bacilli escape into the surrounding space. The meningeal reaction is especially prominent at the base of the brain, where it obstructs the flow of cerebrospinal fluid and entraps the blood vessels. This causes hydrocephalus to develop and reduces the blood supply to the brain itself. If there is no treatment, the pressure in the cranium increases and blood supply stops. For treatment to be effective the illness must be recognized and treated early – before there are signs of damage to the brain.

Diagnosis is always urgent. The illness usually comes on gradually over days or weeks. The condition must always be considered when a previously happy child becomes irritable. The child may complain of headache or have attacks of vomiting. In young children there is often a change in behaviour. Loss of weight is often seen when examining the child's growth chart.

Look particularly for resistance to flexing the neck forwards. Flexing the knee and hip and then trying to extend the knee with the hip flexed often results in the child extending his or her neck and back. Both these are signs of 'meningism', suggesting the possibility of meningitis, which may be tuberculous. Look for signs of cranial nerve lesions, such as squint (from sixth nerve paralysis) or weakness on one side of the face or one side of the body. Look for evidence of tuberculosis elsewhere in the body, including an enlarged spleen which might suggest miliary tuberculosis.

Tuberculous meningitis often complicates disseminated tuberculosis, so that a chest X-ray (if available) can be very helpful to show the presence of miliary tuberculosis. So can examination of the retina with an ophthalmoscope if available. Dilate the pupils first. The presence of choroidal tubercles is diagnostic.

If the disease remains undiagnosed, the child becomes more and more irritable and less responsive, wanting only to lie undisturbed. At that stage he or she often lies curled up on one side. The final stage is when the child fails to respond to any rousing and lies on their back with stiff outstretched legs. From that stage there is little or no hope of recovery. The best hope is therefore to see the child in the early stages. Unfortunately, however, infants are often only brought to the doctor when they are in coma.

If you suspect tuberculous meningitis, when possible send the child to a hospital where X-ray, lumbar puncture and laboratory examination can be done. Details of laboratory findings and diagnosis from other forms of meningitis are given in the section on tuberculous meningitis in adults (page 104).

If transfer is not possible and tuberculosis is suspected, start treatment as soon as possible, as delaying treatment will lead to further brain damage. If prednisone is available, add 2 mg/kg to the treatment as this can reduce brain damage.

Three children with tuberculous meningitis

Severe case: good recovery

Six weeks before admission to hospital, the girl Inez, aged 20 months, had an attack of gastroenteritis with loose stools and vomiting. She improved as the acute symptoms disappeared but she did not regain her normal health. Early one morning 3 weeks later she vomited and did so again several times the same day. For the next few days she was irritable and restless. She cried intermittently, particularly at night, when she would wake screaming. As time went on she grew steadily more irritable. In the 3 days before admission, she had been difficult to rouse.

Inez had received a BCG vaccination at 2 months of age. Shortly afterwards her mother had also been found to have tuberculosis and had been admitted to hospital.

On admission Inez was febrile (39°C), drowsy when left alone, irritable when handled. She had lost weight, there was marked stiffness of the neck and back. X-ray of the chest showed a segmental lesion in the left lower lobe and early calcification in the lymph nodes at the left hilum. The cerebrospinal fluid contained 199 lymphocytes per mm^3 and 140 mg protein%. No TB were seen on direct smear but they were later cultured.

Treatment was started immediately. During the first 10 days Inez's condition did not change. On the 15th day she had twitching movements of her face and irregular jerking movements of the arms and legs. These convulsions were controlled with the use of anticonvulsants. For 2 months more she lay quiet unless disturbed. Over time she seemed to become aware of her surroundings for increasing periods. She began to recognize her name. After 3 months of treatment she was using words and in the next 3 months she learned to sit up, then stand and finally to walk. At that time her cerebrospinal fluid was normal. After that she made an uninterrupted recovery.

A child with tuberculosis of the submandibular lymph node followed by meningitis

Camilla, aged 6 years, had toothache. She then developed an alveolar abscess with a painful swelling of the submandibular lymph node draining the area. The tooth was removed, and the abscess subsided. However, the lymph node could still be felt, although it was no longer tender. Camilla was not quite well and the swelling of the lymph node became larger.

Two weeks later Camilla awoke unusually early and vomited. The next day she was rather irritable and vomited again. She then complained of headache and it was obvious she was losing weight. On the seventh day

cont'd ▶

of that episode she was sent to hospital with the clinical diagnosis of early tuberculous meningitis.

On examination she was thin, rather quiet and anxious, but quite alert and responsive. Stiffness of both the neck and back were found. In the left submandibular area there was an ulcer with a granulating base and thin undermined edges. The adjacent lymph nodes were firm and discrete. At the site of the tooth extraction there was a painless abscess about 2.5 cm in diameter. TB were found in the discharge from the abscess. In the surrounding mucous membrane there were several small 1 mm yellow-grey nodules. The spleen was palpable but no other abnormal physical signs were found.

Lumbar puncture showed a cloudy fluid with 300 lymphocytes per mm^3 and 160 mg protein%.

Treatment was started and Camilla immediately began to improve. The signs of meningitis subsided. Within 2 weeks the lesions in the mouth began to heal. Clinical recovery was complete. Later X-ray showed calcification at the site of the mandibular abscess.

Tuberculous meningitis following another infection and failure to take preventive chemotherapy

Dewi was the second of three sisters, one 2 years older and the other 2 years younger than her. She was 4½ years old when the whole family, including her parents, had an acute infective illness with both cough and loose stools. She was the only one who did not recover quickly. She remained vaguely ill and irritable and vomited occasionally for about a week. She was then brought to hospital. On questioning, the doctor found that about a year earlier her father had been discovered to have chronic pulmonary tuberculosis and had been treated. The children had all been examined. Their X-rays showed that Dewi and her elder sister each had a primary complex in the lung. At that time the children appeared to be in good health but, because of the X-ray findings, they were given chemotherapy. The parents did not accept this, however, and treatment was irregular and ceased entirely after about 3 months.

On examination at the hospital Dewi had a headache, her words were slurred and her neck was stiff. No choroidal tubercles were seen. On lumbar puncture the cerebrospinal fluid was cloudy with 170 mg protein% and 960 cells per mm^3. TB were seen on direct smear and later cultured.

Dewi had been previously treated with isoniazid and ethambutol given together. So the doctor presumed the organisms were still sensitive. She was treated with isoniazid, rifampicin and pyrazinamide, to which streptomycin was added for the first 2 months. She made a rapid recovery.

Tuberculoma

Tuberculous deposits in the brain may become larger without rupturing or causing meningitis. The signs they cause depend on where they are in the brain and the tracts they involve. As they increase in size they have the same effect as a brain tumour. The onset of symptoms and signs is usually slow. Any cranial nerve may be involved, or the child may slowly develop a hemiplegia. In countries where tuberculosis is common, any child who presents with the slow onset of signs of a cerebral tumour should be given a trial of anti-tuberculosis treatment if further investigation is not possible.

Tuberculous arachnoiditis and paraplegia

Tuberculosis may attack the covering membrane of the spinal cord. This may be either an extension of meningitis or a separate site of inflammation. The nerves entering or leaving the spinal cord can be caught up in the process. The spinal cord itself can be compressed, leading to stiffness or paralysis of the legs (paraplegia). The same symptoms may be due to tuberculosis of the spine with the formation of an abscess that compresses the cord. You can easily recognize this if you can obtain an X-ray of the spine. Disease in the spine may be clinically evident as the presence of an angular deformity of the spine produced by the collapse of the bodies of the vertebrae (*Figure 2.12*).

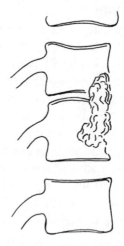

Figure 2.12 *Tuberculosis of the spine:* Diagram of X-ray. Note destruction of adjacent vertebrae and loss of disc space.

Tuberculosis of bones and joints

TB can spread from the primary complex to any bone or joint. The risk that this will happen is greater the younger the child. Most bone or joint disease occurs within 3 years of the first infection but may occur later. Although any bone or joint may be involved, larger weight-bearing joints are most likely to be affected. The spine is most frequently affected, then, with variations in different countries, the hip, the knee, and the bones of the foot, the arm or hand. Swellings in joints come on slowly without the heat and acute pain of a septic infection (though when you lay your hand on it, the joint is often a little warmer than the unaffected joint in the other limb). The slow onset of a swelling over either a bone or a joint should make you think of tuberculosis.

As the clinical pictures are similar in adults and children, these will be dealt with together in this section.

The spine

How it arises
This arises from blood spread of TB. The absence, or narrowing, of the disc space is a characteristic of tuberculosis of the spine. In about 70% of patients, two vertebral bodies are affected; three or more in 20% of patients. The bone lesions are frequently seen in the anterior superior (upper front) or inferior (lower) angle of the body, often with involvement of the adjacent vertebra. As the disease progresses, an abscess forms and this may track to sites such as the lower thoracic cage or below the inguinal (groin) ligament (psoas abscess). It may also compress the spinal cord. The commonest site is the tenth thoracic vertebrae (T10). Frequency decreases the further the vertebra is from T10.

How it presents in the patient
Tuberculosis of the spine is rarely seen in the first year of life. It begins to appear after the child has learnt to walk and jump. After that it may occur at any age.

▶ The first symptom is pain. To reduce the pain, the child or adult holds the back stiffly. The child refuses to bend to pick anything from the floor. If asked to do so, the child may bend at the knees, keeping the back straight. The pain gets better with rest.

▶ Signs differ according to the vertebrae affected.
  – *In the neck.* If the cervical vertebrae are involved, the patient may not like to turn the head, and may sit with the chin propped up by the hand. The patient may feel pain in the neck or shoulders. If an abscess tracks, a soft fluctuant swelling may appear on either side of the neck behind the sternomastoid muscle or bulge into the back of the mouth (pharynx).
  – *In the back down to the last rib (thoracic region).* With disease in that region the patient has a stiff back. When turning, the patient moves the feet rather than swinging from the hips. When picking up something from the floor, the patient bends the knees while the back remains stiff. Later there may be a visible lump or bend in the spine (gibbus), showing where the vertebral bodies have collapsed *(Figure 2.13).*
  – *If the abscess tracks* it may pass to the right or the left around the chest and appear as a soft swelling on the chest wall. (A similar cold abscess can be due to tuberculosis of intercostals lymph nodes.) If it presses to the back it compresses the spinal cord, resulting in paralysis and paraplegia.

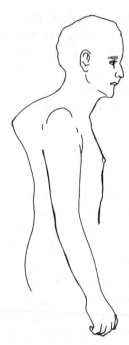

Figure 2.13 *Tuberculosis of the spine: 'gibbus'* – the appearance of a hump or lump in spine due to collapse of vertebral bodies.

- *Lumbar region.* When the spine is affected lower than the chest (lumbar region), the abscess is also below the spinal cord but the pus can track in muscles just as it did at higher levels. If this happens, the abscess may appear as a soft swelling either above or below the ligament in the groin or lower still on the inside of the thigh ('psoas abscess'). Rarely, the pus can track through the opening in the pelvis and reach the surface behind the hip joint. Where tuberculosis is prevalent, perhaps 1 in 4 patients with spinal tuberculosis has a clinically palpable abscess.
- In malnourished patients there may be fever (sometimes high fever), loss of weight and loss of appetite.
▶ In advanced disease there may be not only a gibbus (angulation of the spine) but also weakness of the lower limbs and paralysis (paraplegia) due to pressure on the spinal cord or its blood vessels.

Investigations
▶ If possible, get anterio-posterior and lateral X-rays. The common early features are loss of anterior superior or inferior angle of the body and loss of disc space (Figure 2.12). Remember that multiple lesions may be present in about 10% of patients. A local abscess erodes the anterior surface of the

bodies. An intrathoracic abscess may give rise to an appearance resembling an aortic aneurysm.

▶ Blood tests for typhoid, paratyphoid and brucellosis titres may help in difficult cases at well-equipped centres.

▶ Needle biopsy may also be useful in difficult cases but requires experience and access to good histology.

▶ If the abscess is superficial, you may drain it, else do not attempt to open it. It will subside with treatment.

Complications

The main complication is weakness or paralysis of the legs. Loss of power is sometimes very rapid. If treated quickly, it often responds well (in contrast to paralysis due to tumour etc.).

Differential diagnosis

In most cases the diagnosis is straightforward but tuberculosis may be confused with:

▶ pyogenic infections (e.g. staphylococcal)
▶ enteric infections (e.g. typhoid, paratyphoid)
▶ brucellosis
▶ tumours.

The X-ray appearances are usually characteristic. Evidence of new bone formation (sclerosis) would suggest pyogenic infection. Preservation of vertebral disc suggests a tumour.

An adult with spinal tuberculosis complicated by paraplegia

Ms Fraga, a 48-year-old woman, complained of backache for several weeks. She went to her family doctor who told her that she had lumbago and told her to rest and apply local heat. The pain improved for a week or two, but became worse and began to keep her awake. Her family doctor sent her to hospital where she was X-rayed. The X-ray of the spine was reported to show disease in the 9th and 10th thoracic vertebrae and a malignant tumour was diagnosed. Because primary tumour of the spine is rare, however, her chest was X-rayed and showed almost complete collapse of the left lower lobe. The diagnosis was then changed to primary tumour of the bronchus with secondary tumour in the spine. Radiotherapy was recommended. The following day she developed strange feelings in the legs and began to lose power in them (paraplegia).

cont'd ▶

The same day a physician who specialized in tuberculosis saw Ms Fraga. He pointed out that the X-ray of the spine showed partial collapse of the vertebrae and loss of joint space, and that this was much more likely to be caused by tuberculosis. He recommended that she be examined by bronchoscope. She was found to have a large piece of tuberculous tissue from a lymph node obstructing the left lower lobe bronchus.

The physician immediately began chemotherapy and Ms Fraga made a full recovery.

Comment: Remember that tuberculosis affects all age groups – even those in whom cancer is more common. If there are facilities for investigation, use them to arrive at the right diagnosis; don't jump to conclusions. If diagnosed early, treatment of paraplegia (leg paralysis) due to tuberculosis of the spine is usually very successful – but not if the paralysis is due to a tumour.

The hip

This is the second commonest place for tuberculosis affecting the skeleton. It is more common after 5 years of age.

Young children may just become miserable, stop walking and refuse to walk if asked. Older children and adults may limp and may complain of pain which is sometimes referred to the knee. The limp is due to both pain and muscle spasm. If the condition is not recognized and treated, the joint may be destroyed and the leg shortened.

If possible, watch while the child is playing or moving about so that any limp can be seen. The child is best examined while lying flat on the back on a flat bench or table or even on the floor. It may not be easy to get the child to do this if they are afraid or very young, and patience is required. But if the child will lie with the legs extended, gentle rolling of each leg will detect any spasm in the affected side. You must make sure that the child is lying flat and not with the lumbar region arched forward – slip your hand under the back to make sure. Any arching hides forward flexion of the hip. If the condition is advanced there may be shortening on the affected side. The thigh muscles are usually wasted (smaller). With a tape measure (or piece of string) compare the circumference with the normal side.

If possible, X-ray films should be taken of both hips. Most disease begins inside the joint capsule but occasionally the joint appears clear and the disease is in the neck of the femur. First there is narrowing of the joint space between the acetabulum and the head of the femur but later there are changes in bone as the disease extends. In advanced cases the joint may be destroyed and the femur dislocated.

The slow onset, the results of the clinical examination and the X-ray, if available, should be sufficient to make the diagnosis and to start treatment. At the beginning the child should be at rest until the spasm disappears. The younger the child, the greater the amount of bone regeneration that can be expected; in all children persistence with anti-tuberculosis treatment will bring a great measure of healing.

The history is sufficient to separate tuberculous arthritis from the acute, toxic and painful septic arthritis.

A child with tuberculosis of the hip following a fall

Kadi, aged 9 years, returned home one day and said he had fallen on his right leg. There was no obvious injury and next day he appeared well. About a month later he began to drag that leg and complained of pain in the groin. This limited his movement and he walked with a limp.

On examination there was some wasting of the right thigh. All movements of the right hip were restricted, particularly abduction (outward movement). Kadi's elder sister had had pulmonary tuberculosis for 2 years. Chest X-ray showed a healing primary lesion in Kadi's right lung. X-ray of the right hip showed narrowing of the joint space and some erosion of the acetabulum (the hip socket).

Kadi was put on bed rest and began chemotherapy. Within a few days there was less muscle spasm. After 2 weeks joint movement was almost normal. He went on to make a complete recovery.

The knee joint

Disease in this joint usually begins slowly with swelling, followed by pain, although swelling may be the only sign. The swelling is due to fluid in the joint. The joint is often a little warmer than the unaffected knee. Sometimes there is less fluid, but thickened of the synovium (covering of the joint) may be felt above the patella (knee cap). Compare it with the other knee. The thigh muscles are usually wasted (smaller). In these cases, bone changes may not be found if an X-ray is taken.

In other cases the first evidence of infection may be in the lower part of the femur or the upper part of the tibia, and the changes in the joint are secondary to those in the bone.

The ankle and small bones of the foot

As in other weight-bearing joints, pain and limp are early signs. Swelling over the affected bone or joint indicates the formation of an abscess. The calf muscles are often wasted (smaller). More than one lesion can be present and the same bones may be affected on each side. As in most tuberculosis of bone, the swelling responds well to treatment. If the skin over the swollen area becomes red and fluctuant, draw off the pus with a syringe. This may prevent a discharging sinus.

The arm and hand

The arms are less likely to be affected than the legs. Pain is less likely to be a complaint because weight bearing is less.

In the shoulder, elbow and wrist there is first some limitation of movement and then swelling about the joint. When the small bones of the wrist or the fingers are affected the lesions may be in the same bones on both sides. Tuberculosis of the fingers (dactylitis) may show as an extended, somewhat oval, swelling of the finger, with less swelling round the proximal and terminal phalanges. Several fingers may be affected in each hand. (Infants with sickle cell anaemia may develop dactylitis but this is much more painful.)

As with other large joints, disease in the shoulder can begin either with an effusion into the joint or a bone focus in the head of the humerus; as movement is limited, the muscles of the shoulder girdle become soft and wasted. Tuberculosis of the elbow joint follows the same pattern of reduction in movement, followed by swelling of the joint. Since pain is so much less than with tuberculosis of the bones of the leg, a child may not be seen until there is considerable destruction of the bone.

The first sign of tuberculosis infection of the wrist is nearly always a painless swelling over the back of the hand.

A young child with tuberculosis of the elbow joint

Lamek was first seen when he was 2½ years old. Until he was aged 6 months he had been in frequent contact with an aunt who then died of pulmonary tuberculosis. He seemed to remain well for 2 years. Then his left elbow joint became stiff and movement was limited.

On examination he did not appear generally ill. The left elbow joint was swollen and all movements except pronation were limited. X-ray of the elbow joint showed gross bone destruction in the lower part of the humerus and upper ulna. There was marked loss of the joint surface of the ulna.

The doctor immobilized the elbow in a sling and started chemotherapy. Lamek soon improved. Within 18 months there was good restoration of bone outline. The range of movement steadily increased as the joint was used and Lamek finally achieved an almost full range of movement.

Other bones

Although the bones of the spine and limbs are most often affected, tuberculosis may appear in any bone. It usually shows as a painless swelling. This can slowly become red and discharge, leaving a sinus. More than one swelling may be present.

Occasionally multiple bone abscesses may be seen, usually accompanied by fever. Though most are painless, we have seen painful and tender abscesses in adults, though with little redness of the skin.

X-ray films will show loss of bone shadowing at the site of the swelling.

Cystic tuberculosis of bone

This unusual type of bone tuberculosis needs special attention because it is so different from the sort described above. It is found in areas where tuberculosis is common and has been reported frequently in Africa. It appears as one or more painless swellings which affect the overlying skin to discharge or form abscesses. This appearance is most often found in the hands or feet but it can also appear over the skull or in the long bones, particularly in the head of the humerus near the shoulder joint or in the head of the tibia. X-ray shows that the swelling has cyst-like spaces, with their walls giving a web-like appearance. These cysts are filled with caseating material and contain large numbers of TB. Full treatment is required.

Tuberculosis of the eye

Tuberculosis affects the eyes more often than is realized. Bacilli can be lodged in the eye under the eyelids by dust or by the coughing of an infected person. The bacilli can also reach the eye through blood spread from a primary focus.

Another painful condition – phlyctenular conjunctivitis – occurs which is not due to direct infection but is probably a result of 'sensitivity' to the tuberculin that is being produced at the site of a primary focus in the chest or other site.

Primary infection of the eye (conjunctiva)

If TB lodge under the upper or lower eyelid of a child who has not so far had a primary infection in the lung or abdomen, they can multiply and form a tuberculous lesion. This is the same as a primary infection anywhere else. Multiplication is followed by caseation. You will find small yellow areas if you turn the inner surface of the eyelid outwards.

This reaction does not cause the child much pain or difficulty. The eye may water and be rather irritable, and the lid may become rather swollen. But as the process in the eye develops, the lymph drainage from the area passes to the small lymph node just in front of the ear. This becomes involved in the tuberculous process, enlarges and may soften. It may be the swelling or softening, or even the rupture of the nodal abscess, which brings the child to seek help.

This is a good example of the fact that the first infection with tuberculosis always has both a place of entry of the bacilli and enlargement of the nearest lymph node.

From this type of infection bacilli can also escape into the bloodstream and be carried to other tissues such as bones, just as they can from a primary infection in the lung. The treatment is the same as for primary infection at any site.

Phlyctenular conjunctivitis

This painful reaction can occur at any time following tuberculous infection, but is most common in the first year. It begins with pain, irritation, lachrymation (tears) and photophobia (unwillingness to face light) in one or both eyes. One or more small grey or yellow spots are found round the limbus where the cornea meets the white of the eye. A number of small blood vessels run up from the edge of the conjunctival sac to meet the spots. Each spot lasts about a week and then slowly disappears, but may be replaced by others. In severe attacks the cornea may become ulcerated. Then pain is severe and the patient cannot bear light and shades or closes his or her eyes or sits in the dark.

If secondary infection should follow, there may be a purulent discharge and the cornea may be permanently scarred with white spots where the ulcers had formed.

This painful and sometimes repeated condition is most likely to occur between the age of 5 and 15 years and is common in Africa, India and Southeast Asia. It is usually due to tuberculosis, but can occur with infection by haemolytic streptococci.

Treatment

The pupil should be kept dilated with 0.25% atropine ointment; if there is no sign of secondary infection, 1% hydrocortisone drops will quickly bring relief; however, this cannot be used if infection is present or there is corneal ulceration. Continue the treatment of the primary infection.

Choroidal (retinal) tubercles (Figure 2.14)

Search of the retina with an ophthalmoscope after the pupil has been dilated with 0.25% atropine ointment may sometimes establish the diagnosis of tuberculosis.

The examination is particularly worth doing when rapid diagnosis is required in cases of disseminated disease or tuberculous meningitis. In an ill, irritable child, it may be only possible to examine the retina thoroughly if the child is anaesthetized but this is well worthwhile in a difficult case.

As you look into the eye, note the optic disc and the central artery of the retina which spreads out from its centre. Try to follow each of the main branches in turn as they spread into the retina. If tubercles are present and recent they appear as 1–3 mm yellowish, rounded, slightly raised spots. The edges fade into the general pinkness of the retina. They are most likely to be found within two disc diameters of the centre of the optic disc. As the tubercle gets older the edge becomes more definite and the centre white.

If treatment begins when the tubercle is still yellow, the tubercle can disappear entirely without leaving any scar; if it is white with a sharp edge when first seen, this does not happen and the white area may slowly become filled with black pigmented dots.

Acute tuberculous panophthalmitis

This is a highly destructive abscess of the whole eye. The patient loses vision progressively and the whole of the eye becomes cloudy. Removal of the eye may eventually be necessary.

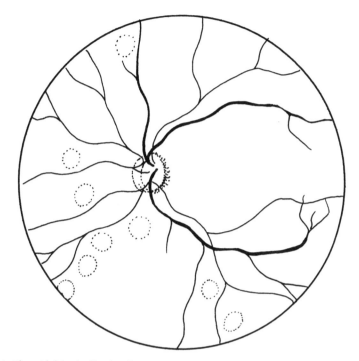

Figure 2.14 *Choroidal (retinal) tubercles.*

Uveitis

'Mutton fat' lesions may occur on the back of the cornea and iris.

Retinitis

Greyish-white ground-glass blotches appear on the retina and the veins may be swollen with local haemorrhages.

Treatment of tuberculosis of the eye

All of the above respond well to treatment with anti-tuberculosis medications. Corticosteroid drugs (if available) can also be valuable in the early stages of destructive disease that threatens the sight or loss of the eye.

Tuberculosis of the skin

Tuberculosis can affect the skin both at the stage of primary infection and during the time when bacilli are spreading in the bloodstream. Primary infections are said to be rare or at least uncommon but, as they are not painful and are often small, it is likely that many are missed.

Primary infection of the skin

Bacilli may enter the skin through a recent cut or abrasion. This most often happens on exposed surfaces. The face, the lower leg and the foot are most commonly affected. The hands and arms are affected much less often.

The original cut or abrasion heals at first. It may then slowly break down over a period of time to form a shallow ulcer. Meanwhile, you see a group of enlarged superficial lymph nodes; you must look carefully in the area that they drain, and suspect any small painless lesion you find. The focus is usually small and may be in the scar of the original wound or abrasion. It may appear like a thickening of the skin and be surrounded by tiny yellowish spots also set in the skin. If the infection has been there for some months before the regional nodes have softened, the focus may have healed to give a central area of smooth scar with a sharply defined irregular edge. The tiny yellow areas will have left sharply defined little bits.

A similar appearance may sometimes be seen in the scar at the site of a BCG infection, as this also produces a primary skin infection.

Abscesses

Two types of tuberculous abscess occur in addition to those that might come from lymph nodes or bones.

▶ The first appears as a soft swelling just under the skin. More than one may be present in different parts of the body at the same time. Being just under the skin, they soon rupture to form an ulcer which usually has a very irregular edge and a clean base. If the child's nutrition is good the ulcers slowly heal. But remember that the child may have other tuberculosis lesions.

▶ The other type of abscess can follow an intra-muscular injection. It is deeper and larger than those described above. Since they follow an injection they are found in injection sites, mostly on the buttocks but sometimes on the outside of the thigh or arm. If the infection results from a dirty needle, and the child has not previously had a primary infection, then the regional lymph nodes are also enlarged and the child may develop tuberculosis in other organs.

Single large painless skin lesions

These are sometimes seen on the hand or face and are set deeply in the skin. Small at first, they can reach 2.5–5 cm and become covered with scaly rough skin. Usually they remain unchanged for months, before slowly healing to leave a scar through the thickness of the skin.

Erythema nodosum and other types of tuberculous skin disease

These are covered in the section on cutaneous tuberculosis in adults (page 116).

Unusual sites of tuberculosis in children

The genital tract

Primary infection

In areas or countries where male circumcision is done as a matter of custom, infection of the wound with TB has occasionally been recorded. When this happens, the wound may heal at first but then breaks down to form the primary focus. The lymph from it drains to the nodes in the groin – usually both sides. These then enlarge and may form abscesses.

Any circumcision wound that does not heal and is followed by enlargement of the nodes on one or both sides should therefore raise the suspicion of tuberculosis.

When the operation is carried out in infants the risk of blood spread and the development of miliary disease or meningitis is high.

Similar risks must arise following genital mutilation of girls ('female circumcision'), when a local lesion and node swelling would develop, although the risk of blood spread varies depends on the age of the child.

Blood-spread disease

In boys before puberty the epididymis just above the testis may become swollen and hard at first. The lump may later soften and discharge through the skin. In young children it is usually only one of a number of lesions in a blood-spread disease. In older boys the testis alone or both the testis and epididymis are more likely to be affected; both enlarge and become attached to the skin and if not treated can soften and discharge.

The process is slow, chronic and relatively painless: it is quite different from an acute bacterial infection with fever, pain, swelling and tenderness of the testis. This is usually part of a urinary infection.

In young girls, tubercles can occur in the uterus and Fallopian tubes as part of the blood spread after primary infection in the lung. These organs can also be involved in tuberculosis of the abdominal cavity following the rupture of a mesenteric node after a primary infection of the intestinal tract. However, pelvic tuberculosis with disease in the uterus or the Fallopian tubes is most usually caused by blood spread from a pulmonary primary infection which has occurred after puberty when the blood supply to the pelvic organs is so much increased. This is important because even if it does not cause symptoms of local disease at the time, it can cause infertility in later years. For this reason many doctors give preventive therapy with isoniazid to tuberculin-positive girls without symptoms.

If disease does develop, the symptoms are lower abdominal pain, loss of weight or appetite, sometimes with lower abdominal distension and amenorrhoea. On examination a mass may be felt in the pelvis, either centrally or to one side. There may be signs of tuberculosis elsewhere in the body. If possible, get an X-ray of the chest.

Treatment should be started as soon as possible; the response is usually good.

The kidneys

Tuberculosis of the urinary system is not often seen in children because it usually develops 7–10 years after the primary infection (see Figure 2.10, page 35).

The infection reaches the kidney via the bloodstream. It develops slowly, beginning between the pyramid and the cortex of the kidney and causing caseation just as it does in the lung. Usually the slow extension opens into the pelvis of the kidney and caseous material is carried in the urine down to the bladder, which may also become diseased. The symptoms of disease may be slight unless the bladder is involved, evidenced by frequent passing of urine and sometimes pain. If there is apparent cystitis, with pus in the urine, but the urine is sterile on culture, remember the possibility of tuberculosis.

When blood is passed in the urine without a complaint of pain, tuberculosis should always be considered and the patient sent where investigation is possible. Of course blood in the urine is common in areas where there is bilharzia (schistosoma). But remember the possibility of tuberculosis. The treatment of all primary infections so that blood spread of bacilli is made harmless would greatly reduce the incidence of renal tuberculosis or rule it out completely.

Tuberculosis of the renal and urinary tracts is covered in more detail in the section on tuberculosis in adults (Section 4.7, page 109). Tuberculosis of the female and male genital tracts is described in Sections 4.8 (page 112) and 4.9 (page 113), respectively.

The liver and spleen

After primary infection, when bacilli are spreading, both the liver and the spleen may become enlarged. This is most marked in young children when the blood spread is heavy (disseminated tuberculosis). But there are many other causes of enlarged liver and spleen. Always consider the whole clinical picture.

Primary infection can occur in the liver of a fetus from the mother (see section below).

Tuberculous of the pericardium

See Section 4.4 (page 106).

Infection before (congenital) or during birth or in the newborn period

Infection can occur if TB passes through the placenta from the mother's circulation into the fetal circulation. Babies can also be infected during or immediately after birth by the inhalation of infected material, or from a birth attendant or other person who has active pulmonary tuberculosis and positive sputum. If a child was infected before birth, the mother must have had tuberculosis during pregnancy and the TB will have reached the fetus through the mother's blood. The mother must have had either a recent primary infection or progressive disease. During a recent primary infection there is often a period when bacilli pass into the bloodstream.

Bacilli that pass through the placenta and enter the fetal circulation are carried by the umbilical veins to the liver. Most of the infants seem well at birth but by about the third week the baby stops gaining weight and becomes jaundiced, with pale stools and dark urine. The liver and spleen are found to be enlarged. The infant has obstructive jaundice because there is a primary focus in the liver and large lymph nodes obstruct the outflow of bile at the porta hepatis. Other causes of jaundice at this period should be excluded.

Sometimes organisms pass through the ductus venosus so that the heart and lungs are the site of infection. If the child has been infected during or immediately after birth, the illness does not become apparent for 3–4 weeks and then quickly resembles an acute pneumonia. The first signs may be attacks of cyanosis or a cough, but the illness worsens rapidly and fine moist sounds can be heard on both sides of the chest. If an X-ray is taken there are inflammatory changes on both sides, often thought to be an acute pneumonia. The only hope is to consider the possibility of tuberculosis and examine stomach washings. Tuberculosis bacilli are usually numerous. The tuberculin test is negative. As soon as diagnosis is made, full treatment must be given. A number of children have recovered.

Chapter 6 provides guidance on the care of the newborn child of a mother with tuberculosis. Of course you should treat any pregnant mother who has tuberculosis, both for her own sake and for the baby's sake. Avoid streptomycin during pregnancy, however, which can cause deafness in the infant.

2.4 How you can help and treat children with tuberculosis

When the child's history, symptoms and physical signs and chest X-ray suggest that the child has tuberculosis you must make a series of decisions.

▶ If a National Tuberculosis Programme policy is laid down for you, then you should comply with it. See that your patient comes under the care of that programme as soon as possible. Local conditions vary and they will of course affect your decisions.

▶ If you must initiate and supervise the child's care and treatment yourself, it will help you to think of four needs:
  – the drugs (chemotherapy) required for tuberculosis
  – medicine required for other infections or infestations
  – attention to the child's nutrition
  – protection against infections that may reduce resistance to tuberculosis.

You should consider each of these aspects of help separately.

Anti-tuberculosis medicines

The immediate action you will have to take when you suspect a child has tuberculosis will depend on the situation in which you are working. There are many variations but they can be summarized into these major categories.

▶ When you are able to, transport or send the child and the family to a larger hospital or tuberculosis centre where the child may be investigated further and treated if necessary. If you send children and their families to other centres, find out later what happens to them.

▶ When the child is so ill that transport to a larger centre is not wise, you must make the decision to start treatment immediately. This applies to children with extensive pulmonary involvement, meningitis or disseminated tuberculosis. On transfer to a larger centre you would send full clinical notes and X-rays with the child.

▶ When you must treat the child yourself, follow the course prescribed for children in your National Tuberculosis Programme. Also pay attention to the important aspects of care described later in this section.

If your National Programme does not lay down a schedule of treatment, you might be limited by the supply of drugs you have available or can obtain. The following approach is flexible, however, and will allow you to do your best whatever your circumstances.

Children who require drug treatment fall into several clinical groups.

▶ *For young children (less than 5 years) without symptoms* of illness who are known to have had a recent primary tuberculosis infection or who have been exposed to a newly diagnosed smear-positive adult with tuberculosis, the objective is to remove the risk of disseminated lesions and to kill the TB in the primary focus and regional nodes of the complex. The treatment should rely on isoniazid 5 mg/kg once daily for up to 9 months.

You may find other children without evidence of disease but with a strongly positive tuberculin reaction. You may not know when they developed the primary infection. Because of the risk of blood spread in young children (less than 5 years of age), most agree that these should be treated with isoniazid alone (as above).

A children of any age who is HIV-positive is at great risk of developing tuberculosis once infected. To reduce this risk, any HIV-infected child who has a positive tuberculin skin test must receive isoniazid (5 mg/kg/day) for 9 months once active tuberculosis has been excluded. The risk is lower at older ages and those who are not HIV-positive; what you do in this situation should depend on the recommendations of your National Programme, your local facilities (e.g. drug supplies) and the circumstances of the particular child.

▶ *Children with symptoms who have pulmonary or extra-pulmonary disease,* such as bone or joint tuberculosis, should be treated according to your National Tuberculosis Programme. The WHO recommends a 6-month regimen with isoniazid and rifampicin, together with pyrazinamide for the first 2 months (doses given in Table 6.3, page 142). Give the drugs in a single dose a day. In several African countries the above regimen is given for the first 2 months only, followed by isoniazid and ethambutol in a single dose a day for 6 months (8 months' treatment in all). However, paediatricians in many countries are reluctant to treat preschool children with ethambutol because of the perceived risk of visual impairment (see below).

▶ *Children who are seriously ill with extensive pulmonary disease*, disseminated tuberculosis or tuberculous meningitis require urgent treatment. You should start treatment at once. If there is no guidance from your National Tuberculosis Programme, treat as above, but add either ethambutol or streptomycin for the first 2 months. For further details of treatment for tuberculous meningitis, see Chapter 6.

Watch the patient carefully for improvement. The first signs may be that the child becomes more aware, and better able to take food and drink. The temperature may begin to come down.

Important note

▶ In the past many paediatricians have used isoniazid at a dose of 10 mg/kg. Neither the WHO nor The Union recommends this.

▶ We no longer recommend using streptomycin for children. This is for three reasons: streptomycin injections are painful; there is a risk of spreading HIV unless syringes can be careful sterilized; and provision of syringes adds to the cost.

▶ Ethambutol at a dose of 20 mg/kg/day (range 15–20 mg/kg/day) has been shown not to cause visual impairment in children, and can be used in children of all ages.

▶ The side-effects of drugs are given in Chapter 6 on treatment.

Multidrug-resistant tuberculosis (see Chapter 6)

Children can be infected with multidrug-resistant TB (bacilli that are resistant to both isoniazid and rifampicin) as easily as with drug-susceptible TB. Multidrug-resistant tuberculosis presents with the same clinical problems as drug-susceptible tuberculosis. Multidrug-resistant tuberculosis should be suspected in a child who has been in contact with an adult known to have multidrug-resistant tuberculosis or who is not responding to treatment while being compliant or an adult who requires retreatment. Children not responding to treatment should also be suspected of having multidrug-resistant tuberculosis. If multidrug-resistant tuberculosis is suspected, refer the child to the local multidrug-resistant tuberculosis expert, as the diagnosis and treatment of multidrug-resistant tuberculosis in children is complex.

Other points in treatment

You may meet a child with a primary infection who does not appear to be ill but you judge needs treatment with preventive isoniazid. It is understandable that the parents may be unwilling to give the child medicine when they cannot see that she or he is ill. Explain the reason slowly and carefully, and give clear answers to their questions. Can you find a parallel in nature where you do something to kill a pest on plants or in animals before they can do harm, rather than waiting for the signs of disease? After all, prophylactic (preventive) medicine is only difficult to accept because they cannot see the thing you are treating. And of course they may not believe the germ theory of disease.

When a child is being treated for tuberculosis, she or he will often soon feel much better, put on weight and become more active well before the treatment is finished. The parents may think that they can then stop the treatment. Explain that the purpose of the treatment is not only to stop the growth of and kill the bacilli, but also to heal the damage the TB have done. The patient feels better but when the medicine is stopped the bacilli start to grow again. The medicine must be continued while the body slowly heals the area where the bacilli have been or allows bone to grow normally again.

Always use a weight chart to show weight change in relation to treatment.

Other medicines

When you treat a child for tuberculosis you must not forget that they may also have other conditions (infective or otherwise) that may need treatment. This, of course, will also help in the general recovery of the patient's health.

In areas where parasites are frequent you should examine the child for these and treat if necessary. Malaria is only one example.

Worm infections, ascaris, hookworm and tapeworms vary in their frequency from one place to another. You will know what is common in your district. Treat any infestation you find.

Children may also have evidence of other infections. The most common are those of the upper respiratory tract, with nasal discharge and obstruction and possibly discharge from one or both ears. If one or both ears are discharging you should try, if possible, to find out whether the discharge contains any TB.

In your examination you may also find that the child has ulcers, pustules or boils. Protect these and treat locally. Also give an antibiotic that is effective against the commonest organisms: staphylococci and streptococci. Skin sores or ulcers may also become infected with diphtheria.

Anaemia, secondary to insufficient intake of iron or to blood loss, is common. You should check the child's haemoglobin as part of the first examination. Correct anaemia with ferrous sulfate tablets (200 mg ferrous sulfate). The correct doses are half a tablet twice daily for infants; 1 tablet twice daily for children aged 2–5 years; 1 tablet three times daily for school-aged children.

Always treat attacks of diarrhoea promptly and with care. Teach parents about oral rehydration and encourage feeding. They should use simple methods (spoon or cup). Make sure they know how to make sugar and salt solution or how to use packets of oral rehydration salts (UNICEF and the WHO). If possible, dissolve these in clean water – boiled if necessary. But boiled water takes a long time to cool. If the child is desperately ill, use the cleanest available water.

Food and nutrition

Tuberculosis and malnutrition travel hand in hand. Tuberculosis causes loss of weight and wasting; insufficient food increases the risk of tuberculosis among those infected with TB and then the spread of tuberculosis. You must always think of nutrition and food with the same care and concern that you think of tuberculosis itself, and of the dangers of other infective illnesses. You must remember that they affect each other.

When you examine a child, always look for signs of malnutrition. Weigh the child and enter the weight on the growth chart. Look at the child's behaviour. Does the child seem hungry or apathetic? Check the quality of hair and skin. Look for skin rash. Is there normal subcutaneous fat? Is there oedema of the feet? From this you will form a first impression of the state of nutrition and whether the situation is urgent.

Decide whether to admit the child to hospital for special observation and treatment. This will include educating the parents, particularly in how to help with the urgent job of improving the child's nutrition.

A child who is very ill and malnourished may be unwilling to take food. Offer small amounts of food often. Nasogastric drip may be necessary until some appetite returns. In countries where milk is part of the diet, this can be used as follows. At first milk (cows', goats', dried or evaporated) can be used with added sugar (50 g or 10 teaspoonfuls to the litre). In severe cases give half-strength feeds every 2 hours to reduce the risk of diarrhoea. Continue for about 3 days, after which high-energy milk feeds can be used. These are prepared by adding vegetable oils to the milk feed and are valuable because they provide extra energy. (Consult your books on the nursing and care of malnourished children. The pocket book *Hospital Care for Children* published by the WHO is a useful reference.)

When the child's appetite returns, begin to introduce the usual local foods to replace the high-energy milk. The mother should always be involved in this care which, for her, will be useful education.

All malnourished children should be given a multivitamin preparation daily. Also give a single dose of 200 000 units of vitamin A in oil by mouth on one occasion, to prevent eye complications.

An ill malnourished child easily becomes hypothermic (low temperature). Hypothermia is very dangerous and further reduces the body's defences. Make sure the child is nursed in a warm place. Mother's warm skin is the best source of heat. Make cotton wool hat and bootees to cover head and feet.

Immunization and protection

Measles and whooping cough may lower the immunity, and the former may increase the risk of tuberculosis. Spread of tuberculosis may occur after a child with a primary infection has had either of these common illnesses. Whenever you treat a child for any form of tuberculosis, you should check his or her clinical history and immunization state.

It there is no reasonable evidence that the child has been immunized or has previously had measles or whooping cough, do all you can to see that he or she is brought into the WHO Expanded Programme on Immunization.

You should be familiar with the immunization policy that is followed in your area and should check as far as possible that all children under your care are protected. Record all immunizations that you give. Also record them on a card for the parents to keep.

Points to remember

Tuberculosis in children can easily be missed, and often is, but you will not miss it if you always keep it in your mind. Always remember the four questions set out at the beginning of this chapter (page 23).

In children, you must think of tuberculosis as a general disease which may appear in any part of the body – not with cough and sputum (which may be blood stained) as is usual in adults.

In children it is difficult to prove the diagnosis by finding TB. This does not mean that you should not try, but it does mean that you must not delay treatment when your clinical judgement tells you that tuberculosis is likely. This may be either because the illness fits into one of those described under question 3 or because a chronic condition in the chest, lymph nodes, a bone or joint, in the abdomen or elsewhere has failed to respond to other treatments.

When you treat tuberculosis in a child, the child's condition and behaviour usually improve quickly. Listen carefully to what the mother says. She is often the first to notice a change. Train yourself to look carefully at your patients as persons as well as at the complaint or symptom that brought them to you. Whoever they are, they need to feel that you care about them.

2.5 HIV infection, AIDS and tuberculosis in children

HIV infection continues to spread rapidly in many countries, especially in sub-Saharan Africa and Southeast Asia. Many women of reproductive age are infected and give birth to infected babies. Immune deficiency due to HIV is now responsible for many hospital admissions. It is a major cause of death of infants in some countries.

Where infection comes from

The most common route of infection is from mother to child during pregnancy or at birth. The risk of an infected mother passing on HIV to her child is between 20 and 40%.

Breastfeeding is an important route of infection with HIV. Whether HIV-infected mothers should breastfeed is therefore controversial. Some say that this should never been done, while others think that breastfeeding is of great importance for the survival of the child. If formula feeding is not possible for socioeconomic reasons or because safe water is not available, then exclusive breastfeeding is advised for 6 months. No other food or water should be given to the baby during this period.

Blood transfusions are a possible source of infection when blood cannot be screened for HIV antibodies. Even where blood is screened, there must be strict rules for transfusion when HIV infection is common in the population. This is because a donor who has been infected recently may give blood before tests can detect antibodies. Few children are infected by blood transfusions.

Contaminated syringes and needles are another possible route of infection.

Diagnosis

The HIV antibody test is unreliable in the diagnosis of HIV infection in children younger than 18 months. The infected mother's antibodies cross the placenta during pregnancy, such that almost all babies born to HIV-positive mothers have HIV antibodies in their blood at birth. Most uninfected babies lose their maternal HIV antibodies by 18 months of age. Most infected babies go on to produce their own antibodies, so in them the antibody test remains positive after 18 months. So, in babies under 18 months it is best to diagnose by clinical signs and symptoms in the baby and a positive HIV antibody test in the mother. If available, a test for the virus itself (not the antibodies) indicates infection in children younger than 18 months. In children older than 18 months the antibody test indicates HIV infection.

Age when children become ill

A few infected babies become ill in the first weeks of life. HIV infection causes one of two clinical pictures in children. Some children have rapid progression of disease (rapid progressors), presenting in the first few months of life with symptoms of severe disease and opportunistic infections. Most of the children in this group die before they are 2 years old if antiretroviral drugs are not available. In the other group of children (slow progressors) the symptoms and signs are delayed for years. Progress is usually more rapid in children than adults. We do not yet know what factors influence the age at which AIDS develops, but tuberculosis allows the virus to multiply more quickly and so speeds progression to AIDS.

Ways in which HIV infection presents in children

HIV infection in children may present with a wide variety of clinical problems. This means that the disease is difficult to define clinically. It can be confused with other diseases. AIDS most commonly presents with a fever, cough, failure to thrive, chronic diarrhoea and itchy rash. Suspect HIV infection when the child has a combination of the signs and symptoms listed below.

Common symptoms

▶ Weight loss or abnormally slow growth
▶ Chronic diarrhoea for more than 1 month
▶ Prolonged fever for more than 1 month
▶ Generalized enlargement of lymph nodes
▶ Thrush (fungal infection) in mouth and throat
▶ Recurrent common infections (e.g. ear infections, pharyngitis)
▶ Persistent cough
▶ Generalized rash

Other common manifestations

▶ Neurological problems
▶ Delay in development
▶ Enlargement of parotid glands on both sides
▶ Enlarged spleen
▶ Enlarged liver
▶ Recurrent abscesses
▶ Meningitis
▶ Herpes simplex

When a child is diagnosed with HIV infection, clinical staging is performed to determine the degree of immune suppression and when antiretroviral drugs should be started. The WHO clinical staging system defines four stages for children: stage 1 is the absence of symptoms or signs of immune suppression; stage 4 indicates severe disease.

It is important to ask about the mother's and father's health. The mother might know her HIV status from being tested in pregnancy. Examine the mother if possible. General enlargement of lymph nodes in the mother or scars of herpes zoster (shingles) can be a useful clue to the diagnosis.

Differentiation from other diseases

Tuberculosis, malnutrition and chronic diarrhoea are common childhood problems in the developing world, and all three are common in HIV-infected children. Several features are common to tuberculosis and HIV infection. These include failure to thrive, loss of weight, intermittent fever, chronic cough, enlargement of liver or spleen, and history of recurrent illnesses. General enlargement of the lymph nodes is rarer with tuberculosis but more common in children with HIV. Chest X-rays may appear similar. Because of reduced immunity, the tuberculin test is often negative in a child who has both HIV infection and tuberculosis.

Prognosis

The prognosis varies with the age when AIDS develops. Children belonging to the rapid progressor group stop growing and suffer frequent infections before they are 1 year old. They often deteriorate and then die in the second or third year of life if not given antiretroviral drugs. Children with slow progression develop symptoms for the first time in their second or third year. These children often continue to grow well despite frequent minor illnesses. If the child has poor nutrition as well as HIV the child is even more vulnerable to fatal infections.

Tuberculosis in HIV-infected children

The natural history of tuberculosis in an HIV-infected child depends on the stage of the HIV infection. If the HIV infection is not yet clinically evident and the child still has good immunity, we can expect the same signs of tuberculosis as in an uninfected child. In an HIV-infected child, however, tuberculosis is more likely to spread to other parts of the body, resulting in tuberculous meningitis, miliary tuberculosis and general enlargement of lymph nodes. The overlap in symptoms and signs between tuberculosis and HIV infection means that the diagnosis of tuberculosis in a HIV-infected child can be difficult. For this reason, always consider the possibility of tuberculosis in an HIV-infected child.

Children who are HIV infected are at great risk of developing tuberculosis. Thus, all children diagnosed with HIV infection must be screened for tuberculosis. If they are found to be infected on the basis of a positive tuberculin test but do not have active disease, this latent infection should be treated with isoniazid (5 mg/kg/day) for 9 months. The decision to treat a child should be considered carefully; once started, the full course of isoniazid must be completed.

Lymphocytic interstitial pneumonia can be particularly difficult to distinguish from miliary tuberculosis in HIV-infected children. Chronic cough, weight loss and fever can occur with both diseases and both can be associated with generalized lymphadenopathy and enlarged liver and spleen. The X-ray pictures are also very similar, both presenting with small widespread nodules. Lymphocytic interstitial pneumonia should be suspected if the child's fingers are clubbed and there is enlargement of the parotid glands. Miliary tuberculosis should be suspected if the child is very ill and has central nervous system involvement.

HIV-infected children usually respond well to anti-tuberculosis drug treatment. When symptoms are suggestive of tuberculosis and the tests to diagnose tuberculosis are inconclusive, it is always worth trying chemotherapy. You must watch the child carefully, and weigh him/her frequently to determine whether there is a response to treatment.

When treating an HIV-infected child for tuberculosis, care should be taken to ensure that the child continues to receive co-trimoxazole prophylaxis, and that immunizations are given.

If the child responds to treatment, try to arrange for him to continue treatment at home. Avoid lengthy hospital admissions, as this exposes these children with little immunity to many risks of infection. It also disrupts family life. Do not use streptomycin injections, as these are painful and increase the risk of spreading HIV infection. Remember also that these children may have other treatable infections.

Counselling

When you suspect that a child may be infected with HIV, it is important to counsel the mother and obtain her consent before you test her blood. When you tell a mother that you suspect her child might have HIV infection, you are giving her very bad news. Her child may have an incurable and fatal disease. She may be infected herself. Her husband may be infected. Any future babies may also be infected.

Try to give her plenty of time to understand, and to ask questions. Discuss the possible advantages and disadvantages of a test for her. If she knows that she is HIV infected she will be able to make important decisions about the future. On the other hand, she may fear that her husband will leave her if she has a positive result. Always ask the mother whether she would like to bring her husband for counselling before she has the test. A woman may find it easier to tell her husband about the possibility of HIV infection than to tell him afterwards that she has had a positive result.

Parents also need counselling when the results are known. Advise them about the outlook for the child and the risk for future babies. Explain how HIV infection spreads. Encourage the parents to change any behaviour that may put other people at risk. Parents will need continued support and counselling to help them to come to terms with the bad news. Common reactions include shock, anger, guilt, grief and depression. It is helpful to train nurses or other health workers in HIV counselling so that they can give enough time to this important aspect of management.

HIV infection and BCG

There have been reports of disseminated BCG in children who have HIV-related suppression of their immunity. In an uninfected child the immune system limits the BCG infection. But in the immune-suppressed child the bacilli can occasionally cause disease.

The WHO recommends that children with known HIV infection should not receive BCG. HIV infection is difficult to diagnose in the newborn. A newborn infant may be HIV seropositive because it has received antibodies, but not virus, from its mother. The WHO recommends that, before giving BCG to the well infant of an HIV-infected mother, careful consideration be given to the risk of developing tuberculosis in that particular country depending on its epidemiological status.

If BCG dissemination does occur, it can be successfully treated with rifampicin and isoniazid. As BCG originally came from a bovine strain, it is resistant to pyrazinamide. Although the BCG dissemination may be controlled, unfortunately the infant is likely to die from AIDS.

Antiretroviral therapy

HIV-infected children respond well to antiretroviral therapy. With the roll out of antiretroviral therapy in the developing world, more children will be started on antiretroviral therapy. A problem arises, however, when the children require treatment for both tuberculosis and HIV. Rifampicin and some of the antiretroviral therapy drugs interact and lower the blood concentration of the antiretroviral drug, rendering the treatment ineffective. The drugs' side-effects can also be confusing. In HIV-infected children the treatment of tuberculosis takes priority and the antiretroviral therapy is delayed for as long as possible – depending on the clinical state of the child and the degree of immune suppression, the antiretroviral therapy can be delayed for 2–8 weeks or until the initial phase of tuberculosis treatment is complete. In HIV-infected children who are not severely immune suppressed, the tuberculosis treatment is completed before starting antiretroviral therapy.

A so-called immune reconstitution inflammatory syndrome (IRIS) has been observed in HIV-infected children being treated for both HIV and tuberculosis. Children who develop this syndrome do so in the first 3–6 months of antiretroviral therapy. IRIS is characterized by clinical deterioration after an initial improvement. The reaction is normally self-limiting, lasting for 10–40 days. Anti-tuberculosis treatment should be continued during this period, but the child may require treatment in a hospital.

If a child is already receiving antiretroviral therapy when the tuberculosis is diagnosed, careful review of the possible drug interactions should be considered and the treatment adjusted accordingly.

Conclusions

Tuberculosis in children can easily be missed – and often is – but you will not miss it if you always keep the possibility in mind. Always remember the four questions set out at the beginning of this chapter (page 23).

In children you must think of tuberculosis as a generalized disease that may appear in any part of the body – not necessarily with cough and sputum (which may be blood stained) as is usual in adults. The ways it presents is described in Section 2.3.

In children it is difficult to prove the diagnosis by finding TB. This does not mean that you should not try, but it does mean that you must not delay treatment when your clinical judgement tells you that tuberculosis is likely. This may be either because the illness fits into one of those described under question 3, or because a chronic condition in the chest, lymph nodes, a bone or joint, in the abdomen or elsewhere has failed to respond to other treatments.

When you diagnose tuberculosis in a child, always consider that the child could be co-infected with HIV; counsel the mother and do the HIV test.

When you treat tuberculosis in a child, the child's condition and behaviour usually improve quickly. Listen carefully to what the mother says. She is often the first to notice a change. Train yourself to look carefully at your patients as people as well as at the complaint or symptom that brought them to you. Whoever they are, they need to feel that you care about them.

Chapter 3
Pulmonary tuberculosis in adults

3.1 Pulmonary tuberculosis

How pulmonary tuberculosis develops in adults

In Chapter 2 we described how lung lesions might arise from the primary lesion in a child. Here we describe what may happen in adults. In an adult, pulmonary (lung) tuberculosis may arise in a number of ways.

▶ *Progression of a primary lung infection in a person who has never previously been infected* (previously tuberculin negative). In progressive primary tuberculosis in adults, the mid and lower parts of the lung are involved more frequently than the upper lung zones.

▶ *Progression of lung lesions comes from the blood spread of bacilli*, which normally occurs after a primary lesion. These bacilli may end up in the lung as in other organs (*Figure 3.1*). If there are many bacilli and defences are poor, disseminated tuberculosis results. If there are only a few bacilli and defences are good, the bacilli may be killed. In between, lesions may start at one or both apices of the lung and later spread to other areas. This is an uncommon way for adult tuberculosis to develop.

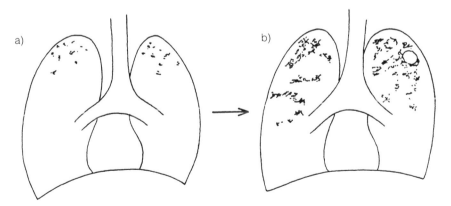

Figure 3.1 *X-ray appearance of the blood spread of some types of pulmonary tuberculosis.* a) Blood spread of TB from the primary lesion (invisible) to form small lesions at the apex of each lung. Higher oxygen in this part of the lungs encourages the growth of the bacilli. b) Lesions have become confluent (run together). A cavity has developed on the left. Disease has spread to the mid zone of each lung.

▶ *Reactivation of an earlier primary infection,* perhaps years after a childhood infection by TB *(Figure 3.2a–d).* The patient's defences may have kept the lesion under control in childhood, but lowering of the patient's defences (e.g. by malnutrition, pregnancy, parturition or other diseases) may allow the TB to become active and spread the disease. In post-primary tuberculosis, the lesion is often in the apex or upper zone of the lung. The lung lesion is often more obvious than the lymph node enlargement, which you may not be able to detect on an X-ray. This is a common way for tuberculosis to develop in adults.

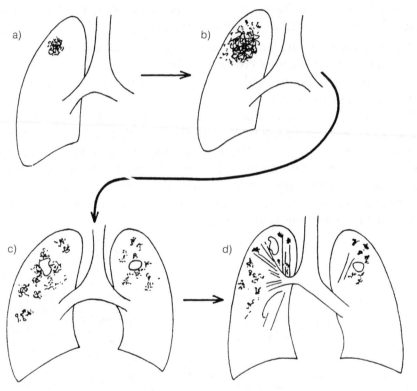

Figure 3.2 *X-ray appearances of post-primary tuberculosis in an adult.* a) The primary lung lesion in an adult is often in the upper part of the lung. The lesion in the hilar lymph node is often not visible on the X-ray (though the nodes may be greatly enlarged in a patient with HIV infection). The lung and lymph node lesions often heal and may later calcify. But there may be: b) gradual enlargement of the lung lesion; c) caseation of the lesion. Liquefied caseous material may be coughed up, which results in a cavity. Spread of TB from the cavity produces further lesions in either lung (with a further cavity developing in that lung). d) After a year or two (if the patient survives), the development of fibrosis (scarring) can pull up the right hilum and pull the trachea over to the right. Calcification is starting in older apical lesions. Note the cavities are still open. This type of 'chronic survivor' is a major source of infection.

▶ *Reactivation of an old post-primary lesion* that had been partially healed.
▶ *Re-infection* may happen in persons previously infected with tuberculosis and progress to disease.

In adults, the lymph node components (hilar or paratracheal) of the primary complex are usually not visible in an X-ray, although they may be very prominent in a patient with HIV infection; and the patient sometimes has high fever. In patients with HIV infection, tuberculous enlargement of hilar or paratracheal nodes may sometimes occur months or years after the primary infection.

In adults, tuberculous lesions occur particularly in the upper parts of the lungs because the oxygen level is higher there; this helps the TB to grow.

Spread within the lung often results from the caseation (cheesy necrosis) in the lesion, followed by breakdown into liquid material. The liquid material is coughed up, leaving an air-containing cavity. TB multiply rapidly in the cavity and can spread through the bronchi to new areas of lung. Lesions may be patchy, or they may join together to form tuberculous pneumonia. This may again break down into further cavities.

The lesions may heal by fibrosis or scar tissue, or there can be a mixture, with worsening in some areas and fibrosis occurring at the same time in others. Some lesions may calcify, showing as white material on the X-ray. Later the fibrosis may shrink so that, on the X-ray, the hilar shadows are pulled up or the trachea pulled over to that side. The lesions may damage the walls of the bronchi and produce bronchiectasis, with gross widening of the bronchi. As the bronchiectasis is usually in the upper lobes and is well drained by gravity, mostly it does not cause symptoms itself (apart from the symptoms of tuberculosis).

Identifying the adult who might have pulmonary tuberculosis

Most cases of pulmonary tuberculosis are diagnosed as the result of the patient feeling unwell and so coming for help to a health centre, clinic, hospital or private doctor.

Cough and sputum is very common everywhere. Much of this is due to acute respiratory infections and usually lasts 1–2 weeks. Chronic cough is frequently associated with chronic obstructive pulmonary disease. This is mostly due to tobacco smoking, but may also occur from atmospheric pollution (inside buildings, from cooking or heating fires, or outside, from air pollution). As we shall see, certain additional symptoms may suggest tuberculosis. But often this is not obvious: the only way to make sure is to examine the sputum for TB in anyone who has had a cough for 3 weeks or longer.

Here follow some guidelines as to how you can best make the diagnosis of pulmonary tuberculosis. The symptoms and signs are described below.

<table>
<tr><td colspan="2">Symptoms (see also Figure 1.3, page 13)</td></tr>
<tr><td>

Respiratory
- • • Cough
- • • Sputum
- • • Coughing up blood-stained sputum
- • Chest wall pain
- • Breathlessness
- • Localized wheeze
- • Frequent colds

</td><td>

General
- • • Loss of weight
- • • Fever and sweating
- • Tiredness
- • Loss of appetite

</td></tr>
</table>

The number of dots shows which symptoms are most important.

Note that all the symptoms could be due to other illnesses. To make sure, you must examine the sputum for TB.

Some patients may come to a clinic shortly after the onset of symptoms. They may have only a cough. Patients who come late usually have more symptoms. The type of symptoms you observe among your patients and how frequently they occur depend partly on how soon patients visit your facilities after the onset of symptoms. One of the most important things that should make you think of possible tuberculosis is that the symptoms have come on gradually over weeks or months. This applies particularly to the general symptoms of illness: loss of weight, loss of appetite, tiredness or fever.

Cough, of course, is a common symptom following acute respiratory infections. It is also common in smokers and in some areas where the houses or huts have no chimneys and the houses are often full of smoke – especially in cold climates or cold weather when fires may be used for heating as well as cooking. Both tobacco and domestic smoke lead to chronic bronchitis. Cough may come on gradually in a patient with lung cancer, which is becoming more frequent in countries as cigarette smoking increases. Bronchiectasis is common in some countries: the patient may have had a chronic cough with yellow or green sputum from time to time since childhood. But if a patient has had a cough for more than 3 weeks you must get his or her sputum examined for TB to determine whether the cough is due to tuberculosis. The appearance of the sputum may not itself suggest tuberculosis: it may be clear, green or yellow, or it may contain blood. In tuberculosis, blood in the sputum may vary from a few spots to the sudden coughing of a large amount of blood. Occasionally this blood loss is so great that the patient quickly dies, usually from choking on the blood. If you see blood in the sputum you must always examine the sputum for TB.

Pain in the chest is not uncommon in tuberculosis. Sometimes it is just a dull ache. Sometimes it is worse on breathing in (due to pleurisy). Sometimes it is due to muscle strain from coughing. Sometimes the cough is so severe that the patient has cracked a rib (cough fracture).

Breathlessness in tuberculosis is due to extensive disease in the lungs, or to pleural effusion complicating the lung tuberculosis. The breathless patient frequently appears ill and has lost weight and will often have fever.

Occasionally the patient has a localized wheeze. This is due to local tuberculous bronchitis or to pressure of a lymph node on a bronchus.

Sometimes the patient seems to have developed an acute pneumonia but the pneumonia does not get better with routine antibiotics. The cough and fever may persist and the patient remains ill. Do not forget to examine the sputum for TB. If questioned closely, sometimes you may find that the patient reports cough and loss of weight for weeks or months before the pneumonia came on.

Sometimes the patient reports having had one cold after another. When you question carefully, you find that the colds may be just that a chronic cough has gotten repeatedly worse; examine the sputum for TB.

Remember that, in an older smoker, cough and loss of weight that came on gradually may be due to lung cancer. But you must check for tuberculosis by examining the sputum; a patient may have both diseases.

Women who develop tuberculosis may lose their periods (amenorrhoea). They usually have other symptoms as well.

Physical signs

Physical signs do not often help much, but do examine the patient carefully. You may find useful signs.

▶ *General condition.* Sometimes this may be good, in spite of advanced disease. But the patient may be obviously ill: very thin, with obvious loss of weight; pale or have a flush due to fever.

▶ *Fever.* This can be of any type. There may be only a slight rise of temperature in the evening. The temperature may be high or irregular. Often there is no fever.

▶ *Pulse* is usually raised in proportion to fever.

▶ *Finger clubbing* may occur, particularly in a patient with extensive disease. Remember that clubbing is more common with lung cancer, lung abscess or bronchiectasis.

▶ *Chest.* Often there are no abnormal signs. The commonest sign is fine crepitations (crackles) in the upper part of one or both lungs. These are heard particularly on taking a deep breath after coughing. Later there may be dullness to percussion or even bronchial breathing in the upper part of both lungs. Occasionally there is a localized wheeze due to local tuberculous bronchitis or pressure by a lymph node on a bronchus. In chronic tuberculosis with much fibrosis (scarring), the scarring may pull the trachea or the heart over to one side. At any stage the physical signs of pleural effusion may be present. Often, however, you will find nothing abnormal in the chest.

Investigations

Microscopy

The most reliable way of making the diagnosis is to find TB in a direct smear of the sputum. Examination is by the Ziehl–Neelsen staining method or, in a busy and well-equipped centre, by using fluorescence microscopy. The flow chart in *Figure 3.3* is a guide to making the diagnosis.

Remember the following points when collecting sputum for examination.

▶ The container should be rigid to avoid crushing when carried or sent. It should be wide-mouthed and be made of material that can be burnt. It should have a tight-fitting screw top to prevent drying out or leakage.

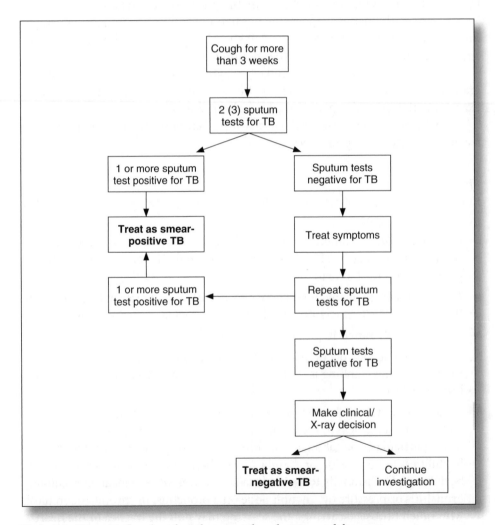

Figure 3.3 *Diagnostic flow chart for pulmonary tuberculosis in an adult suspect.*

▶ Examine at least two specimens if possible:
  – a first spot specimen when the patient first presents
  – an early morning specimen consisting of all the sputum raised in the first 1–2 hours.

▶ Instructions to the technician for collection of sputum:
  – If possible do the procedure in the open air. If not, use a well-ventilated room set aside for this purpose.
  – Explain why the test is important. Explain how to cough so as to produce sputum from deep in the chest.
  – Label the bottom part of the container (not the lid) with the name and number of the patient and give the bottom part to the patient to provide the specimen. Keep the lid.
  – Ask the patient to hold the container close to the lips, then cough and spit into it.
  – Check that the specimen has solid or purulent particles in it. If not, get the patient to try again.
  – Close the container securely. Put it in a special box for the laboratory.
  – Wash your hands thoroughly with soap and water.
  – Keep a full and accurate register of sputum examinations. Make sure the specimens are properly labelled, with the patient's name clearly marked.

Culture

Culture of sputum slightly improves the number of positives, but it may take 4–8 weeks before you get the result. With milder disease and fewer TB, the smears may be negative but culture positive. But culture requires skilled laboratory facilities which you may not have. While waiting for the culture result(s) you will have to decide on the basis of clinical evidence, and X-ray if available, whether or not to start treatment (see Chapter 6). The most ill patients and most severe cases (who most need treatment and who are most infectious) are usually smear positive.

Drug resistance tests

Drug resistance tests can only be done in specialized laboratories. In most developing countries the specialized laboratory is best used to look at the pattern of drug resistance in the community. It should not usually be used to help in the management of individual patients. Find out whether the pattern has been worked out for your own area. In countries with a DOTS-Plus programme, it may be used to identify multidrug-resistant tuberculosis among patients who are at a high risk (such as treatment failure in retreatment cases). These patients can then be offered the more complex and expensive treatment for this type of disease in the centre that provides this care.

Special examinations
The following investigations are possible only in well-equipped specialist centres.

Laryngeal swabs
In patients who do not have sputum, a laboratory that can do cultures may be able to provide you with these special swabs. The operator should wear a mask and gown when taking a swab. The patient's tongue is held using a piece of lint, and the swab pushed down behind the tongue towards the larynx. The patient will cough and the swab will catch some mucus. Put the swab back into the sterile bottle and send to the laboratory for culture.

Gastric aspiration
Gastric aspiration is often called 'gastric lavage' or 'washings'. This may be used when a patient has no sputum. It is only necessary if you have some difficult problem in diagnosis and if you have the facilities. It is sometimes used in children, who seldom produce sputum (Appendix F). In adults, do gastric aspiration soon after the patient wakes and before he has taken anything by mouth. Pass a well-lubricated fine rubber nasogastric tube through the nose to the back of the mouth. Then ask the patient to suck water through a 'straw' or fine tube. While the patient does this, push the nasal tube gently in and it will pass easily into the stomach. Attach a syringe containing 20 ml of sterile normal saline through the nasogastric tube. Inject it slowly down the tube. Wait about a minute and then aspirate as much as possible back into the syringe. Transfer the contents into a sterile bottle and send to the laboratory. There it can be examined by smear and culture.

Bronchoscopy
When other methods have failed to help you make a diagnosis you may be able to collect bronchial material by a trap specimen through a bronchoscope. Biopsy of the lining of the bronchi may sometimes show typical changes of tuberculosis when examined by histology. If you do bronchoscopy for diagnosis of tuberculosis, take extreme caution to avoid becoming infected with TB.

Pleural fluid
TB may occasionally be seen in centrifuged fluid but usually are only found on culture. The larger the amount of fluid cultured, the more likely it is that you will get a positive.

Pleural biopsy
Pleural biopsy can be useful when there is pleural effusion. But it needs a special biopsy needle (such as Abrams punch), facilities for histology and training in the technique. If available, pleural biopsy specimens should be sent for culture, in which case the diagnostic yield is very high. To do this will require that you submit the specimens separately for histology and for culture. In many places none of these is available.

Lung biopsy

Only experienced operators should use this method. A diagnosis may be made by histology or by finding TB in the sections.

X-ray (radiological) examination

You cannot diagnose tuberculosis with certainty from an X-ray, as other diseases often look very similar.

For practical purposes, a normal chest X-ray excludes tuberculosis. Very rarely, however, endobronchial tuberculosis or disease hidden by the mediastinum or diaphragm may look like a normal chest X-ray. Furthermore, HIV-infected patients with tuberculosis are more likely to have a normal chest X-ray.

The following X-ray shadows are strongly suggest of tuberculosis:

▶ upper zone patchy or nodular shadows (on one or both sides), illustrated in Figure 2.1c (page 25) and Figure 3.1a (page 75)
▶ cavitation (particularly if more than one cavity), shown in Figures 3.1b (page 75) and 3.2c (page 76).

Calcified shadows may cause difficulties in diagnosis. Remember that pneumonia and lung tumours can occur in areas of previous healed and calcified tuberculosis. Some benign tumours contain calcification.

Other shadows that may be due to tuberculosis are:

▶ oval or round solitary shadow (tuberculoma) *(Figure 3.4a)*
▶ hilar and mediastinal shadows due to enlarged lymph nodes (persisting primary complex; Figure 3.4b)
▶ diffuse small nodular shadows (miliary tuberculosis; Figure 3.4c).

The correct reading of chest X-rays needs a lot of experience.

If you suspect tuberculosis from the X-ray but the sputum is negative, give a non-tuberculosis antibiotic (e.g. ampicillin, oxytetracyline) for 7–10 days then obtain another X-ray. Shadows of an acute pneumonia will show improvement. But beware of shadows that look smaller after 10 days but are in fact due to collapse of part of the lung resulting from obstruction of a bronchus.

> You must *always* examine the sputum. It is a major error to diagnose tuberculosis from an X-ray but fail to examine the sputum.

Tuberculin test

Technical details of tuberculin testing are given in Appendix E. Although, with proper attention to careful technique, tuberculin testing is very useful in measuring the prevalence of tuberculous infection in a community, it is of limited value in diagnosing active tuberculosis in adults. This is because the test may be negative because of malnutrition or other diseases, even though the patient has

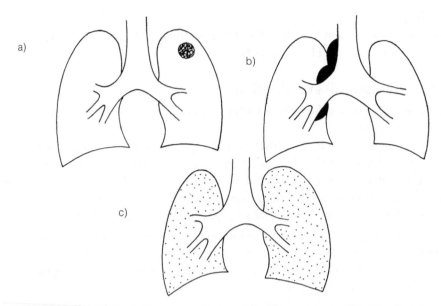

Figure 3.4 *Some further X-ray findings in pulmonary tuberculosis.* a) Rounded 'tuberculoma' or coin lesion in the upper zone of the left lung. b) Enlarged right hilar and paratracheal lymph nodes of the primary complex (may be with or without obvious lung component). In an adult this appearance may look like a hilar carcinoma. Sometimes it is accompanied by high fever. This sort of appearance is very rare in adults of European origin, except in HIV-infected patients, but may occur in adult Asians or Africans. c) The diffuse, evenly distributed, small nodular lesions of miliary tuberculosis. In the earliest stages these may be difficult to detect.

active tuberculosis. A positive test simply indicates tuberculous infection, which is very frequent in many countries and does not indicate the presence of disease. (Remember a strongly positive test is only a point in favour; many people without active tuberculosis have positive tests. In general the test is of little use for adults.)

There are two other problems in using the tuberculin test.

▶ *False positive:* in many countries infection by other, often non-pathogenic, environmental mycobacteria can result in a positive tuberculin test, but usually a weak positive. A positive can also be due to previous BCG.

▶ *False negative:* problems of improper storage, improper dilution, absorption of tuberculin onto glass, contamination etc. may make the test unreliable in your area. We suggest you consult a local tuberculosis specialist, who should be able to tell you whether the test will be valuable in your area.

On the other hand, a positive test, even a strongly positive test, shows only that the patient has previously been infected. It does not prove that he or she has active tuberculosis disease. It is merely a point in favour.

The frequency of positive tests increases with age. A positive test is therefore more meaningful the younger the child is, particularly if not vaccinated with BCG.

> **Important note**
>
> Always remember that a negative test does not exclude tuberculosis; a positive test does not indicate disease.

Blood examination

Marked anaemia is rarely caused by pulmonary tuberculosis but it is sometimes seen in obscure ('cryptic') disseminated tuberculosis. Anaemia is more likely to be due to other causes such as worms or malnutrition.

The white blood cell count is raised in some patients but can be normal or low normal. (It is often raised in pneumonia.)

The erythrocyte sedimentation rate may be raised. But a normal result does not exclude active tuberculosis. This is therefore not a useful test and is not worth doing.

Low serum potassium or sodium may occur in severe disease and can cause death. Many centres will not have facilities for these tests. If found, correct the electrolyte balance by intravenous infusion.

Finally, all patients presenting with cough and sputum for 3 or more weeks must have their sputum examined for TB.

Newer 'molecular' diagnostic methods

Much work is being done on methods to detect molecular components of TB in sputum but so far these are not sufficiently straightforward or reliable for general use. The same applies to blood serum antibody tests. Methods are also being developed for rapid testing of drug resistance.

Distinguishing tuberculosis from other conditions

The main conditions that have to be distinguished are described below.

Pneumonia

The symptoms of acute pneumonia usually come on suddenly. In the X-ray, the abnormal shadows may look like tuberculosis, particularly if they are in the upper part of the lung. If the sputum is negative, give an antibiotic that is not active against TB (e.g. ampicillin, oxytetracyline) for 7 days and X-ray again. A raised white blood cell count is in favour of pneumonia but the count can be normal or low normal in elderly patients with pneumonia. If you have no X-ray, a rapid fall in temperature when you give the antibiotic makes the diagnosis likely to be pneumonia.

Pneumonia due to *Pneumocystis jirovecii* (formerly known as *P. carinii*) is a common disease in advanced HIV infection (AIDS). There is often a low-grade fever for several weeks and cough without sputum. For details, see Chapter 5 on tuberculosis and HIV/AIDS.

Lung cancer

On the X-ray a tumour may sometimes break down into a cavity. Or infection beyond a bronchus blocked by a tumour may cause a lung abscess with a cavity. If the sputum is negative, diagnosis may have to be made by bronchoscopy. A solid rounded tumour may be difficult to distinguish on the X-ray from a rounded tuberculous lesion. A patient with lung cancer commonly is a smoker. Feel also for an enlarged lymph node behind the inner end of the clavicle, a common place for secondary tumour.

Lung abscess

There is usually a lot of purulent sputum and the patient is usually feverish and ill. If the purulent sputum is repeatedly negative for TB, lung abscess is more likely. The white blood cell count is usually high.

Bronchiectasis

There is usually a lot of purulent sputum and it has often been produced since childhood. Persistent coarse 'crackles' may be repeatedly heard over the same area of the lung. Patients with bronchiectasis may develop tuberculosis. When in doubt, check the sputum for TB.

Asthma

Patients with asthma experience episodic wheeze, productive cough, shortness of breath and chest tightness. Wheeze is not common in tuberculosis but it may occasionally occur from:

▶ enlarged lymph nodes, which may obstruct a bronchus or even the trachea
▶ tuberculous bronchitis.

Either of these may cause a localized wheeze. Remember also that a few patients with severe asthma may be on long-term corticosteroid drugs (such as prednisolone). This can weaken the patient's defences against TB, resulting in tuberculosis along with the asthma. If a patient with asthma develops a cough while under treatment, or begins to run a fever or loses weight, test the sputum for TB.

Some stories about diagnosis

A happy story

Ms Kamal, a 20-year-old woman, had recently married and had gone to live with her husband in his parents' house. A few months later she began to feel tired, lost her appetite and began to cough a little. At first the family thought it was the strain of recent marriage. Then stopped her periods and they thought she might be pregnant. In the end her mother-in-law

cont'd ▶

took her to the outpatient department of the district hospital. Her symptoms had now lasted 2 months. The doctor thought tuberculosis was a possibility. He asked if anyone else in the family had a cough. The mother-in-law said that her husband (the patient's father-in-law) had had a chronic cough for a year or more and had lost some weight.

On examination the doctor found Ms Kamal to be rather thin and she had a slight fever. He found nothing else abnormal. He asked her to cough up some sputum into a container. He gave her another container. He asked her to cough into it first thing the next morning, producing as much sputum as she could. He sent her for a chest X-ray.

The doctor asked Ms Kamal and her mother-in-law to come back the next morning with the sputum specimen. He would then tell them about the X-ray result. He asked the mother-in-law to bring her husband at the same time so that he could find out the cause of the husband's cough.

The 'spot specimen' of sputum that Ms Kamal had given in the clinic tested negative. But the early morning sputum she produced next day tested positive for TB. So as to make sure, the doctor asked for another spot sputum sample, which also tested positive. The X-ray showed soft shadows in the right upper zone of the lung, with a small cavity.

The father-in-law's sputum also proved strongly positive on two occasions. His chest X-ray was abnormal. Ms Kamal's husband and her mother-in-law were well. They had no cough and no sputum to test. Their chest X-rays were clear.

The doctor explained everything in a careful and friendly way to the whole family. He told them all about the treatment and gave them each a leaflet to take home. Both patients took their treatment regularly and came back regularly for medicine. Both of them soon lost their symptoms and felt very well.

A year and a half later Ms Kamal presented her husband with a son. The whole family came back to see the doctor and to thank him. The doctor arranged for the new son to receive BCG as a precaution.

A more complicated story – the diagnosis nearly missed

Mr Ram Musa, a 40-year-old man, had been a farm worker. One year ago he had moved with his family to the city in search of a better life. Since then he had worked in a factory. He was paid only a small wage. This was not enough to give his family decent housing. He and his wife and three children lived in a hut he had built on waste ground.

Mr Musa was a heavy smoker. For some years he had had a 'smoker's cough', worse in the morning. For the last 3 months his cough had got

cont'd ▶

worse. He began to feel more tired than usual. His appetite became poorer. He thought he was getting thinner.

He first went to a local healer. The healer gave him medicine and charged him a fee. But Mr Musa got worse, not better. So he went to a private doctor, who gave him an antibiotic and charged him a fee. He went back to the doctor several times. The doctor gave him other medicines and charged him more fees. The patient's condition continued to get worse.

Finally, now feeling very ill and having run out of money, Mr Musa went to a government health centre where there was a well-trained health assistant. Because Mr Musa had a chronic cough, loss of appetite and loss of weight, the health assistant thought he might have tuberculosis. When he examined him he found that he was thin and had a slight fever. There were no definite physical signs in the chest. There was no X-ray machine at the health centre.

The health assistant asked Mr Musa to give a specimen of sputum right away. He gave him another sputum container and asked him to cough into it first thing the next morning and come back to the clinic. Both specimens of sputum tested positive for TB.

The health assistant decided that he would start Mr Musa on anti-tuberculosis chemotherapy right away. In a kind and friendly way he told him the diagnosis and the treatment. He told him how long it would last and why. He gave him a leaflet to remind him of what he had been told. Mr Musa could not read, but his 10-year-old son could and would be able to read the leaflet to him at home.

The health assistant asked Mr Musa to come back the next day with his wife and children. When they came back he greeted them in a friendly way. He told the wife what he had already told the patient. He told them both that if Mr Musa did not take his treatment regularly the tuberculosis might come back and kill him. He also told him that smoking was bad for his health. If he continued smoking, the tuberculosis might come back after cure. He said that if he stopped smoking it would help him to feel better quickly. It would also give him more money to support his family. If he took his treatment regularly he could continue to work, as otherwise the children would starve.

The health assistant examined Mr Musa's wife and children. They felt well. He found nothing obviously wrong. The children had been born in a remote country area and they had not received BCG: there was no scar on any of their arms. The health assistant gave the children and the wife tuberculin tests. He asked them to come back 3 days later when he read the tests. The tests of the 10-year-old boy and the 7-year-

cont'd ▶

old girl were negative. The test of the 3-year-old daughter was strongly positive. Because at that age there is a big risk of the child developing miliary tuberculosis or tuberculous meningitis after a tuberculous primary infection, the health assistant prescribed daily isoniazid for 9 months for this child.

The wife had a weakly positive tuberculin test. He asked her to come back at once if she developed a cough or felt ill in any way.

In any case she came back regularly with the 3-year-old child to get new supplies of isoniazid. The health assistant made sure on each occasion that both the child and the mother seemed well.

Mr Musa soon lost his cough, felt very much better and began to put on weight. He also stopped smoking. Two sputum samples were negative when tested after 2 months' treatment. He was now feeling so much better that he was doing his work at the factory much better. So he was given a better job and got more money. He was also saving money by not smoking. So he was able to move his family into a better home. The child remained well after a year and was discharged from the clinic.

Comment: This is a common story. Mr Musa may have been infected with TB when he came into the town. There he lived in bad conditions and probably met many people with infectious tuberculosis. Or the bad conditions he was living in may have caused an old primary infection to break down.

In many countries patients will first go to local healers. In some places doctors have tried to encourage local healers to send patients to health clinics or health centres if they seem really ill or don't recover quickly. The private doctor should have had the patient's sputum examined for TB. Many private doctors fail to do this: it is very bad medicine.

The health assistant did his job very well. He immediately thought of tuberculosis and had the sputum examined. He gave the right treatment. He took time and trouble to explain everything in a friendly way to both the patient and his wife. He immediately looked for possible tuberculosis in the wife and children. He gave preventive treatment to the youngest child, who had probably been recently infected by her father. He not only cured Mr Musa and his daughter from tuberculosis. He also helped him to stop smoking. So everyone in the family ended up both well and also less poor.

A wrong diagnosis

Mr Koso Bang, a 20-year-old young man, had a smoker's cough. One winter he had a bad cold. The cough got worse and he produced more

cont'd ▶

yellow sputum. After 10 days he went to see a private doctor who sent him for an X-ray. He had to pay a fee for the doctor and he had to pay for the X-ray. The X-ray showed some abnormal shadows in the upper part of the left lung. The doctor diagnosed tuberculosis. He started Mr Bang on treatment with rifampicin and isoniazid. He did not examine the sputum for TB. Mr Bang soon felt rather better. But he only had enough money now to pay for 2 weeks' treatment. He did not have enough money to go back to the doctor. So he went to the outpatient department of the district hospital. There the doctor repeated the X-ray and asked him to produce two specimens of sputum which he had examined for TB. The X-ray was normal. The two sputum samples were negative.

The doctor told Mr Bang that he did not have tuberculosis but a mild pneumonia which had now cleared up. But he strongly advised him to stop smoking. If he did not, he might easily get pneumonia again and could get tuberculosis also. Mr Bang stopped smoking, his cough disappeared completely and he continued to feel well.

Comment: You cannot diagnose tuberculosis with certainty from an X-ray. Pneumonia can look the same. Many patients are caused a lot of anxiety and take unnecessary anti-tuberculosis treatment for many months because a doctor has made a misdiagnosis of tuberculosis from an X-ray and has failed to examine the sputum. You *must* examine the sputum for TB. You may give an antibiotic. If a shadow is due to pneumonia, it will improve or disappear in 2–3 weeks.

A mistaken case of 'pneumonia'

Mr Chowdhuri, a 50-year-old man, was admitted to a district hospital with 'pneumonia'. He had had a bad cough and felt feverish for 7–10 days. For 3 days he had had a pain in the right side of his chest, worse when he breathed in. The doctor found him flushed, ill and obviously breathless. He had a high temperature and a fast pulse. The doctor heard crepitations (crackles) scattered on both sides of the chest. The patient was unable to take a deep breath because of the pain in the right side of his chest; the doctor could not hear the pleural rub. X-ray of the chest showed scattered patches on both sides.

The doctor decided that Mr Chowdhuri had bronchopneumonia and prescribed amoxicillin. After 5 days he was, if anything, worse. The doctor then questioned him carefully about his illness. Mr Chowdhuri said that for several months he had been feeling tired and had lost some weight. He had had a little cough. Ten days before he came into hospital these symptoms had begun to get much worse and he felt very feverish.

cont'd ▶

With this more detailed story, the doctor thought the illnesses could be tuberculosis. He sent three sputum specimens for examination for TB. They came back positive. When the doctor got the results of the sputum tests, he immediately put the patient on anti-tuberculosis chemotherapy. Within a few days there was great improvement. In 10 days the fever had subsided. Soon after that Mr Chowdhuri went home to continue his treatment at a nearby health centre. In due course he recovered completely.

Comment: Occasionally a patient with tuberculosis may seem to have acute pneumonia, but this fails to improve with pneumonia treatment. You must examine the sputum for TB. If you question the patient closely, you will often find that the patient has had some symptoms for weeks or months before these became more acute and brought him to hospital.

Complications

Pleurisy and empyema
These are discussed in Section 3.2 (page 92).

Spontaneous pneumothorax
Spontaneous pneumothorax occurs when air escapes into the pleural space following rupture of a tuberculous cavity or a subpleural caseous focus. This causes sudden acute chest pain on that side, together with breathlessness. It may go on to tuberculous empyema.

Tuberculous laryngitis
This is described in Section 4.1 (page 103).

Cor pulmonale
Cor pulmonale (congestive cardiac failure due to back pressure from a damaged lung) may occur if there is very extensive destruction of the lungs. This may happen even if tuberculosis is no longer active but has left a lot of scarring. Early treatment of tuberculosis obviously makes this less likely.

Aspergilloma
Well treated and 'healed' tuberculous cavities sometimes remain open and can be infected by the fungus *Aspergillus fumigatus*. On the X-ray you may see a ball of fungus within the cavity. This sometimes causes severe, and even fatal, haemoptysis (coughing up blood). If bleeding keeps on recurring, and you have got surgical facilities, you may have to consider resecting the cavity. But often the patient's lung function has been greatly reduced by the damage from the old tuberculosis so that he is not fit for surgery.

3.2 Tuberculous pleural effusion and empyema

How the pleura are affected

The pleura may be affected in three different ways:

▶ effusion that develops within a few months of primary infection in children and young adults

▶ effusion developing as a result of lung disease in older adults; rarely this may go on to a purulent effusion (empyema)

▶ rupture of a tuberculous cavity and escape of air into the pleural space, allowing air to escape into the space between the lung and the chest wall. The TB from the ruptured cavity produces a purulent effusion (empyema). The air and the pus together are called a pyopneumothorax.

Clinical appearance

The following signs and symptoms may be seen:

▶ pain when the patient breathes in (pleuritic pain) which later becomes a dull ache in the lower chest

▶ fever, which may be mild and not last long

▶ slight irritating cough

▶ breathlessness on exertion

▶ dullness to percussion over the lower part of the chest

▶ no sounds of air entry when you listen over that area of the chest

▶ in large effusions, the mediastinum is pushed away from the affected side *(Figure 3.5)*.

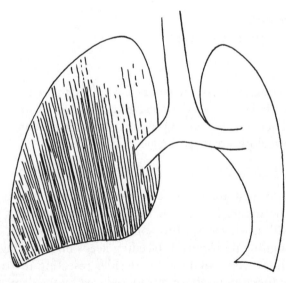

Figure 3.5 *Large right pleural effusion.* Note that the trachea, heart and mediastinum are pushed over to the left.

The tuberculin test is sometimes negative, particularly if the patient is malnourished, has recently had measles or is infected with HIV. If negative at first, the test may prove positive if you repeat it a month later.

There may be an abscess over the lower chest if the empyema spreads through the chest wall between the ribs. Remember that a 'cold' fluctuant swelling – not hot or tender – can be due to a 'cold abscess' from a tuberculous intercostal lymph node or an abscess tracking round the chest wall from a tuberculous spine.

Investigations

X-ray of the chest
Large effusions are most dense at the base, thinner at the top. You cannot see the diaphragm, and the angle between the diaphragm and chest wall is lost. The shadow thins out at the top. If you are not sure whether fluid is present, take another X-ray with the patient lateral decubitus (lying on the lesion side) or supine (lying flat on his back). The fluid shadow will move.

If a cavity has burst, air as well as liquid will be present. The top of the fluid will be flat, with the air above it *(Figure 3.6)*. This gives a splashing sound if you shake the chest.

Removing fluid
Remove some fluid with a syringe and needle (or by intercostal tube if the pus is too thick). Send the fluid or pus for examination for TB.

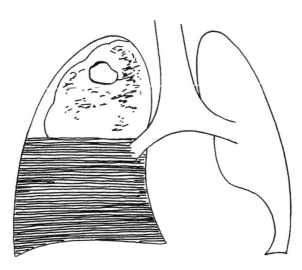

Figure 3.6 *A cavity has burst into the pleura.* Air as well as fluid is present. The top of the fluid will be flat. The fluid often turns to pus (pyopneumothorax).

Removing tissue

If you have the facilities and the training, at the same time remove a piece of pleura tissue (biopsy). Send this for examination under the microscope (histology).

Other conditions that have to be distinguished

▶ Tumour
▶ Other infections (e.g. pneumonia; pleural fluid resulting from amoebic abscess of the liver, if on right side)
▶ Heart disease
▶ Liver disease
▶ Kidney disease
▶ Pulmonary embolism and infarction

Management

▶ Treatment is detailed in Chapter 6.
▶ Aspiration (drawing off) of fluid: this will probably only be required once, and only if the effusion is causing discomfort. There is usually rapid response to treatment with no need for aspiration.
▶ Sometimes it may be necessary to remove a localized empyema surgically.

End result

This is usually satisfactory. But, if neglected, the pleura may become very thick and fibrotic. This can cause shrinkage of the chest wall and later breathlessness.

3.3 Disseminated tuberculosis

How it arises

Disseminated (including miliary) tuberculosis is due to spread through the bloodstream of large numbers of TB that the patient's defences are too weak to kill off. (It is called 'miliary' because the small lesions in the organs seemed to 19th century pathologists to look like millet seeds. The term is now applied when they appear as small rounded shadows on the chest X-ray.) TB may enter the blood by:

▶ spread to the bloodstream from a recent primary infection – this may occur by way of the lymph nodes and lymphatics or by a tuberculous lesion eroding a blood vessel
▶ reactivation of an old tuberculous lesion (post-primary) with erosion of a blood vessel; reactivation may occur if the patient's defences are lowered, for instance by HIV infection, another disease, malnutrition or old age
▶ spread into the bloodstream after surgery on an organ containing a tuberculous lesion (always give chemotherapy before surgery, to reduce the number of TB, and continue treatment after operation to kill all bacilli).

Why diagnosis is particularly important

If not properly treated, almost all patients with disseminated tuberculosis will die. If properly treated, almost all patients should recover. If you can get an X-ray of the chest, the diagnosis may be quite easy, but in some cases it can be very difficult. The X-ray may fail to show the lesions. In some places no X-ray may be available. Moreover, particularly in the elderly, the disease may be much less acute ('cryptic miliary tuberculosis' described below) and it is easy to forget this possibility.

Clinical appearance in adults

Clinically disseminated tuberculosis has traditionally been divided into two different types: classic and cryptic, mainly from the perspective of chest X-ray manifestations *(Table 3.1* overleaf). A third form, which can be termed non-reactive disseminated tuberculosis, occurs in patients who are profoundly immunosuppressed, and is seen in patients with HIV/AIDS.

Classic disseminated tuberculosis

Chest X-ray is the most useful tool in detecting miliary tuberculosis. The clinical presentations are non-specific. Common symptoms include fever, anorexia, weakness, weight loss and cough. The onset of fever and other symptoms can be gradual, usually over weeks, and may follow some other illness (e.g. measles). There is nothing typical about the kind of fever, which varies widely. There may be evidence of a tuberculous lesion somewhere in the body, but often this is not obvious. Sometimes there is enlargement of the liver or spleen (though less often than in children) – but of course there are many other possible reasons for this.

If you have an ophthalmoscope, look for choroidal tubercles (See Figure 2.14, page 59). These are seen less often in adults than in children but if present make the diagnosis certain. Check for neck stiffness and other signs of meningeal irritation – tuberculous meningitis often complicates disseminated tuberculosis.

X-ray of the chest shows small, diffuse, evenly distributed shadows. They vary in different cases from vague shadows 1–2 mm in diameter to large dense shadows 5–10 mm in diameter. The white blood cell count is usually normal or low. The tuberculin test may be negative. Without treatment, death usually follows in weeks, but sometimes after as long as 1–3 months.

Cryptic disseminated tuberculosis

The diagnosis of cryptic (obscure) disseminated tuberculosis may be missed in patients without typical presentation of disseminated tuberculosis; often the correct diagnosis is made only at post mortem. This form of tuberculosis usually occurs in the elderly. The fever is often mild or irregular and may continue over months, and there is often anaemia. There are usually no other helpful physical signs. The illness may not be visible on the chest X-ray. Lesions may only appear

Table 3.1 Summary of types of disseminated tuberculosis in adults			
	Acute 'classic'	Cryptic	'Non-reactive'
Frequency	Common	Rare	Very rare
Age	Any age	Usually elderly	Any age
Fever, malaise, loss of weight	Prominent	Mild	Usually desperately ill
Choroidal tubercles	15–30%	Absent	? Absent
Meningitis	10%	May be terminal	Absent
Enlargement of liver/spleen	May be present	Rare	May be present
Chest X-ray	Usually miliary shadows	No shadows at first	May or may not show shadows
Tuberculin test	Positive or negative	Often negative	Usually negative
Blood abnormality	May be anaemia etc.	Often anaemia	May be anaemia (often aplastic), pancytopenia, agranulocytosis, leukaemoid reaction
Low serum sodium/ potassium	Especially in elderly and women	Normal	?
Diagnostic biopsy	Seldom needed	Often helps	Diagnostic, especially bone marrow

after weeks or months. If you do suspect miliary tuberculosis, shine a bright light behind the outer rib spaces: this may show the first small lesions. The tuberculin test is usually negative. Cryptic meningitis is a frequent cause of pyrexia of unknown origin when tuberculosis is common. Without treatment, the patient's condition gets slowly worse over months and the patient eventually dies, with or without terminal meningitis.

Non-reactive disseminated tuberculosis

A special form of disseminated tuberculosis, which can be termed non-reactive disseminated tuberculosis, happens in patients with profound immunosuppression. Before the HIV epidemic this was very rare. However, it is now not uncommon in HIV-infected patients with a low CD4 count. It is an acute malignant form of tuberculous septicaemia (spread of large numbers of TB through the bloodstream). Histologically (under the microscope) the lesions are necrotic, not typical of tuberculosis (poor granuloma formation with minimal cellular reaction), but with very large numbers of TB. The patient is extremely ill. The chest X-ray may or may not show lesions (also sometimes called cryptic miliary tuberculosis, *Figure 3.7*). The tuberculin test is negative. There are often blood abnormalities. These may include anaemia (often aplastic), pancytopenia (especially leukopenia or agranulocytosis) or appearances similar to leukaemia. The diagnosis is often missed, in which case the patient is likely to die rapidly.

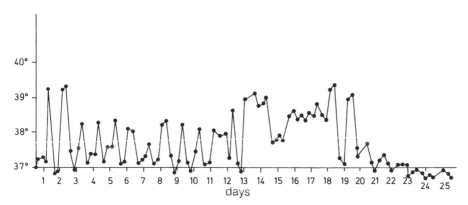

Figure 3.7 *Cryptic disseminated tuberculosis* diagnosed because the patient's condition improved with specific anti-tuberculosis treatment. The man, aged 70 years, had continued fever, anaemia, a negative tuberculin test and no direct evidence of miliary tuberculosis: no abnormal clinical signs and an apparently normal chest X-ray. Usual investigations for fever of unknown origin were negative. Using treatment with para-aminosalicylic acid and isoniazid (which would not affect other infections) his temperature fell and his blood count returned to normal.

Diagnosis of disseminated tuberculosis

Fever
Fever is common in tropical countries and finding the cause is probably one of your most frequent tasks. Make sure you always consider the possibility of disseminated tuberculosis. For your patient it may make the difference between life and death.

Duration of symptoms
If the history suggests that fever has been present for more than 7–10 days (which will exclude most acute infections), you must think of the possibility of disseminated tuberculosis. You must have a routine for investigating fever of unknown origin. Your routine will partly depend on the common causes in your area, and partly on your facilities for investigation (e.g. white blood cell counts, blood cultures and X-ray).

X-ray
A chest X-ray may be virtually diagnostic, if you can get one. Viral or bacterial pneumonia may occasionally look like disseminated (miliary) tuberculosis, but the shadows are likely to improve within a week or so with treatment for pneumonia. But, as we have already pointed out, a normal X-ray does not exclude disseminated tuberculosis.

Sputum smear examination
Sputum smear is usually negative. Culture is of limited use, even if possible, because the result will come back too late to help you. Urine culture may also be positive in due course.

Other specific investigations
These are only needed in a difficult case. If you have the facilities, liver or bone marrow biopsy may show necrotizing granulomas on histology. If possible, make sure part of the specimen is put in a sterile container (i.e. with no preservative, which would kill TB) and sent for culture for TB. The result of culture will arrive too late to influence a decision about treatment but may later confirm your diagnosis.

Response to treatment
If the diagnosis is not clear clinically, if the chest X-ray is negative and you have no other means of diagnosis but you believe the case is one of tuberculosis, start the patient on anti-tuberculosis treatment and register the patient as a case of tuberculosis. If the disease is tuberculosis, the fever will usually begin to come down within a week (Figure 3.7).

Treatment

Disseminated tuberculosis responds well to standard chemotherapy. Fever usually begins to come down and malaise is relieved within days (occasionally longer); it usually takes a month or more before the X-ray starts to clear.

If the patient is desperately ill (with either acute or the rare non-reactive disseminated tuberculosis), and you have the facilities, it is justified to give prednisolone with your chemotherapy. This will reduce the life-threatening toxicity and give the anti-tuberculosis drugs time to act. But it is dangerous to use prednisolone unless you are sure of the diagnosis (in case you are suppressing the patient's defences against some undiagnosed infection you are not treating).

Two stories about disseminated tuberculosis

A man attending a moderately well-equipped district hospital

Mr Wong Fan, an 18-year-old man, came to the outpatient department at a district hospital. He looked very ill. He had a high temperature. He said that he had begun to feel tired about a month before. This had got steadily worse. He felt more and more ill. He felt feverish and sweated a lot. He lost his appetite. He was getting thinner. He had had a slight cough for several weeks, but he had no other symptoms.

Because he looked so ill, the outpatient doctor immediately admitted him to a ward. There, the doctor found a few crepitations (crackles) on each side of the chest. He could just feel the tip of the spleen. There was no neck stiffness, no rash, and no enlarged lymph nodes. The doctor knew that malaria was common in the area, so many patients had an enlarged spleen. The story seemed a long one for typhoid. Miliary tuberculosis must be a possibility. He asked about cough or tuberculosis in the family. The patient said there was none.

To look for evidence of miliary tuberculosis, the doctor dilated the pupils with eye drops. With his ophthalmoscope he carefully searched each retina for choroidal tubercles. He found two small yellowish slightly raised areas near a blood vessel in the left retina. These were typical of choroidal tubercles. This made the diagnosis nearly certain. But he also got an X-ray of the chest. This showed widespread 2–3 mm rounded shadows throughout both lungs.

To be on the safe side, the doctor sent three blood smears for malaria parasites. He also ordered three sputum examinations for TB (culture for TB was not available). The blood smears were negative for malaria. There was very little mucoid sputum; these smears were negative for TB.

cont'd ▶

Because he had found the choroidal tubercles and the patient was very ill, the doctor did not wait for the results of these investigations. He started the patient on anti-tuberculosis chemotherapy straight away.

Mr Wong's temperature began to come down within 3 days. He felt much better and began to eat well. After 10 days the temperature was normal and he was gaining weight. He was then sent home to continue his treatment.

Before Mr Wong left, the doctor carefully explained to him about the disease. He also gave him a leaflet that explained the treatment, and he explained to the family at the same time. He explained to the parents that the patient's life depended on his taking every dose of the treatment for the full time. Otherwise the disease might come back and kill him. While Mr Wong was in hospital the doctor checked his parents and three siblings for tuberculosis: none was found.

Comment: This was a straightforward case. With an ophthalmoscope and an X-ray it was easy to investigate because the doctor thought about tuberculosis, so he looked for choroidal tubercles and then got an X-ray of the chest. But remember that many patients with miliary tuberculosis will not have choroidal tubercles. Remember also that in the early stages miliary shadows may not show on the chest X-ray. Remember that in miliary tuberculosis the sputum is often negative on direct smear. It is often positive on culture. But culture may not be available; in any case you would have to decide about treatment before you got the result.

A woman attending a rural health post with few facilities

Ms Mawi, a married woman aged 23, had been feverish and ill for the last 10 days. She went to a local healer. He gave her medicine but she went on getting worse. She was now so ill that she had to be carried to the health post. She had headache with the fever but no other symptoms: no cough, no urinary symptoms, and no diarrhoea.

The health assistant found that Ms Mawi was thin and ill and had a high temperature. He found nothing abnormal in the chest. He could not feel the spleen or liver. There was no rash and no neck stiffness. He had no ophthalmoscope and had not been trained to use one.

The health assistant examined a blood slide for malaria: it was negative. Three sputum samples were examined for TB and were negative. He thought she might have an enteric infection (typhoid or paratyphoid) or perhaps some other infection or miliary tuberculosis. He asked about tuberculosis or whether any of the family had a chronic cough. They said that everyone else was well. He decided to give chloramphenicol first. This would deal with enteric and some other bacterial infections He could not

cont'd ▶

refer the patient to hospital as the nearest was a day's walk away and there was no road or transport. The patient was obviously not fit to make the journey. Ms Mawi lived close to the health post. Because she was so ill, 3 days later the health assistant went to see her at home. She said she was no better; indeed she was worse. She was now so ill that the health assistant decided that she could wait no longer. He added anti-tuberculosis chemotherapy. To be on the safe side, he also continued chloramphenicol for a further 10 days. He did this in case she had an enteric infection that was slow to improve with treatment. To be on the safe side he also took another blood smear for malaria. This was negative.

The next day the patient was a little better. Three days later she was definitely feeling better and her temperature was lower. She gradually recovered completely. The health assistant carefully explained the importance of taking all the treatment for the full period, even after she was feeling entirely well. He also explained this to the family.

Although the family has said that everyone else was well, when he visited the home the health assistant noticed that the patient's mother-in-law had a cough. She said that she had had this for a year or more, but did not feel ill. The health assistant arranged for three sputum tests for TB. Two of these were positive. So he also successfully treated her.

Ms Mawi's two children, aged 3 and 5, had been given BCG when they were infants. There were BCG scars on their arms. No tuberculin was available. They were well, but clearly had been at major risk of infection so he arranged for them both to have 9 months of preventive isoniazid. He also explained that if they or the husband or the father-in-law became unwell they should come to the health post at one. But all remained well.

Comment: Where there are few facilities, the doctor or health assistant has to do his best with what he has got. He has to look for clues in the patient's story. In particular, ask about family illness that could be tuberculosis. But if you can get no help from the story or physical signs, and if it is not possible to refer the very ill patient to other facilities, you may have to decide to put the patient on anti-tuberculosis treatment. The patient might be getting better from something else on his own. But it is the best you can do.

With this patient, it might have been better to continue the chloramphenicol for a week before deciding that it had failed. But the patient's condition was getting rapidly worse. The health assistant rightly decided that it was too big a risk to wait. So he added anti-tuberculosis treatment. The patient improved rapidly. This made tuberculosis highly probable, although the improvement might have been a delayed effect of the chloramphenicol. But miliary tuberculosis is fatal without proper treatment. So it was much safer to treat it as miliary.

cont'd ▶

Note that the family had denied other illness. But the health assistant was sufficiently alert to spot the mother-in-law's cough. When he found her sputum positive this strongly confirmed the diagnosis in the original patient.

Chapter 4
Extra-pulmonary tuberculosis in adults

4.1 Tuberculosis of the upper respiratory tract

Nearly all tuberculosis of the upper respiratory tract (epiglottis, larynx and pharynx) is a complication of extensive and prolonged pulmonary disease and is usually sputum-smear positive. Blood-borne infection occasionally causes laryngeal tuberculosis with little to find elsewhere. Laryngeal tuberculosis has often been wrongly diagnosed as cancer of the larynx. The epiglottis is often involved in laryngeal tuberculosis. The pharynx may also be affected.

Clinical features

- ▶ The patient may have had cough and sputum for some time, as laryngeal disease occurs most often in advanced pulmonary tuberculosis. They may also have lost weight.
- ▶ There may be hoarseness and changes in the voice, becoming a moist whisper.
- ▶ The patient may have pain in the ear, or pain on swallowing, which usually means the epiglottis is also involved. Pain may be severe.
- ▶ In very advanced disease the tongue may show ulcers.
- ▶ Examination shows ulceration of the cords or other areas in the upper respiratory tract.
- ▶ Examine the sputum for TB, which usually tests positive.
- ▶ X-ray the chest if the sputum smear is negative.

Distinguishing it from other diseases

Cancer is the main disease from which tuberculosis has to be distinguished. Malignant disease of the larynx is rarely painful. The sputum smear is positive in most cases of tuberculosis of the larynx, but the diagnosis may need to be made by biopsy in rare cases.

Management

Tuberculosis of the larynx responds extremely well to chemotherapy. If there is severe pain that does not clear quickly with treatment, add prednisolone for 2–3 weeks (if available).

4.2 Tuberculosis of the mouth, tonsils and tongue

Tuberculosis of the mouth is rare and usually occurs in the gums. It shows as a relatively painless swelling which is often ulcerated. As it is frequently a primary lesion, there is often enlargement of the regional lymph nodes. Both this and tonsillar lesions, which are similar, are likely to be caused by infected milk, or perhaps occasionally food, or infected droplets from the air. Tonsillar lesions may not be obvious clinically.

Lesions of the tongue are usually secondary to advanced pulmonary tuberculosis. They are often ulcerated and may be very painful. They improve rapidly with chemotherapy.

4.3 Tuberculous meningitis

Tuberculous meningitis remains a major problem and an important cause of death in some countries. It occurs more frequently in patients with advanced HIV infection and in these patients may also be caused by environmental mycobacteria.

How it arises

In the course of spread from the primary tuberculous focus, or as part of the spread of disseminated tuberculosis, bacteria are seeded into the brain and meninges, where they form tiny tubercles. Occasionally bacteria may also be seeded into the bones of the skull or the vertebrae. These tubercles may rupture into the subarachnoid space and there cause:

▶ inflammation of the meninges
▶ formation of a grey jelly-like mass at the base of the brain
▶ inflammation and narrowing of the arteries to the brain, which may cause local brain damage.

These three processes cause the clinical picture.

Clinical features

There is usually a history of general ill health for 2–8 weeks – malaise, tiredness, irritability, changes in behaviour, loss of appetite, loss of weight and mild fever. Then, as a result of inflammation of the meninges, there will be headaches, vomiting and neck stiffness. The grey exudates involving the base of the brain may affect the cranial nerves, giving some of the expected signs: deterioration of vision, paralysis of an eyelid, squint, unequal pupils, deafness. Papilloedema is present in 40% of patients. Involvement of the arteries to the brain can lead to fits, loss of speech or loss of power in a limb or limbs. But any area of the brain may be damaged. Some degree of hydrocephalus is common. This is due to blocking by exudates of some of the cerebrospinal fluid connections within the brain. Hydrocephalus is the main reason for decrease of consciousness. The resulting damage may be permanent and probably accounts for the poor prognosis in patients who are only seen when they are already unconscious. Spinal block by exudates may cause upper motor neurone weakness or paralysis of the legs. As tuberculosis is often present elsewhere in the body, look for:

▶ tuberculosis of the lymph nodes
▶ X-ray evidence of lung disease, especially disseminated (miliary) tuberculosis (if X-ray available)
▶ enlargement of liver and/or spleen
▶ (choroidal) tubercles visible on examination of the retina (see Figure 2.14, page 59).

The tuberculin test may be negative, particularly in the advanced stages of the disease.

Diagnosis

The main conditions to be distinguished are:

▶ bacterial meningitis
▶ viral meningitis
▶ HIV-related cryptococcal meningitis.

In the first two of these the onset is much more acute. Cryptococcal meningitis may have a much slower onset. A family history of tuberculosis, or the finding of tuberculosis somewhere else in the body, makes tuberculosis much more likely. But the best evidence comes from examination of the cerebrospinal fluid obtained by lumbar puncture. The points are as follows:

▶ *Cerebrospinal fluid pressure* – usually raised
▶ *Appearance*: at first looks clear but may form a 'spider's web' clot on standing. May be yellowish if there is spinal block.
▶ *Cells*: 200–800 per mm^3. Many neutrophils at first (but not all neutrophils as in bacterial meningitis, which has a much higher cell count). Mainly lymphocytes later. The count may be low in patients with advanced HIV infection/AIDS.
▶ *Glucose*: low in 90% of patients, but may be normal in the early stage of the disease and in patients infected with HIV. This is particularly helpful in differentiating from viral meningitis, in which the glucose is normal.
▶ *Bacteriology*: smear is positive in only 10%, unless a large volume (10–12 ml) is centrifuged long and hard. If the microscopist spends 30 minutes or more on a thick smear slide, then up to 90% positives can be reached. Culture should be carried out if possible. It is usually positive, but can only give late confirmation of your diagnosis. Bacteriological diagnosis may obviously be made by obtaining mycobacteria from other specimens (e.g. sputum, pus). In areas of high HIV infection, do Indian ink stain for cryptococci.

Prognosis

Death is certain if the disease is untreated; disability results if diagnosis and treatment are delayed. The earlier the infection is diagnosed and treated, the more likely the patient is to recover without serious permanent damage. The clearer the state of consciousness when treatment is started, the better is the prognosis. If the patient is comatose, the prognosis for complete recovery is poor. Unfortunately 10–30% of survivors are left with some damage.

Because of the fatal outlook if diagnosis is missed, it is best to treat if the diagnosis is at all likely. Details of treatment are given in Chapter 6.

4.4 Tuberculosis of the pericardium

This is rare in many parts of the world and relatively common in others, especially where HIV infection is widespread.

How it arises

The bacilli may reach the pericardium through the blood (when there may also be disease in other organs). But it is more commonly due to rupture of a mediastinal lymph node into the pericardial space. It is rare for tuberculosis of the lungs to be present at the same time.

Clinical features

Dry pericarditis
Dry pericarditis presents with:

▶ acute pain that the patient feels behind the sternum – it may be relieved by sitting forward
▶ friction rub heard with the stethoscope over the heart and in time with the heart beat
▶ if you can get an electrocardiogram you are likely to see widespread T-wave changes.

When pericardial effusion develops, the clinical signs are:

▶ breathlessness on exertion (or even at rest)
▶ a rapid pulse that is paradoxical: a large fall in blood pressure and pulse pressure on inspiration; this is not always present (this is because normally the negative pressure in the thorax on inspiration draws blood from the great veins into the heart – this is prevented if there is too much fluid in the pericardium)
▶ low blood pressure (sometimes severe)
▶ raised jugular venous pressure
▶ enlarged liver
▶ fluid in the abdomen
▶ fever (of variable degree)
▶ the friction rub may disappear as fluid develops but it sometimes continues.

X-ray examination usually shows a large pericardial effusion (see Figure 2.8, page 30).

Constrictive pericarditis

The inflammation may make the pericardium thicker and even calcified. Calcification may show on the X-ray as a narrow irregular white rim along the edge of the heart shadow *(Figure 4.1)*. The thickened pericardium may form a sort of armour or casing over the heart. This may prevent it dilating in diastole (the expansion of the heart that draws in the blood). The result is that the heart cannot take in enough blood from the veins.

The constriction may occur within months or weeks of the effusion but sometimes it only shows years later, perhaps with no history suggesting a previous pericardial effusion.

The patient may come with the following signs and symptoms.

▶ *Breathlessness* – as the lungs are not congested, the patient can lie down without increased breathlessness. There is no pulmonary oedema so no diffuse pulmonary crepitations.
▶ There is oedema of legs etc., due to back pressure in the systemic veins.
▶ The liver may be very large. There may be ascites. The spleen may be enlarged.
▶ The heart is small and quiet. This is quite different from most causes, or congestive cardiac failure, which is associated with a large heart.
▶ The jugular venous pressure rises with inspiration (whereas normally it would fall).
▶ There is paradoxical pulse (see previous page).

Look for signs of tuberculosis elsewhere in the body.

Most cases of constrictive pericarditis are due to tuberculosis. It is particularly suggested by the small heart, in spite of marked evidence of oedema in the limbs without congestion in the lungs. If possible, take penetrating (black) X-rays which may show up the calcification, confirming the diagnosis.

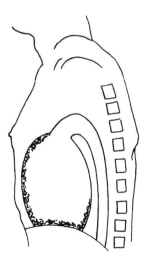

Figure 4.1 *Constrictive pericarditis.* Lateral X-ray film showing thickening and calcification of the pericardium. This 'armour' prevents full dilatation of the heart, compromising its function.

Diagnosis

Diagnosis of tuberculous pericarditis is made by:

▶ evidence of tuberculosis elsewhere in the body
▶ culture of pericardial fluid, if this is possible (60% positive)
▶ biopsy of pericardium, if this is possible (70% positive).

It has to be distinguished from disease of the heart muscles, other causes of heart failure and malignant disease.

A case of tuberculous pericarditis in a 9-year-old boy

Four months previously Tomas had developed erythema nodosum. At that time the doctor thought that this was connected with rheumatic fever. He had been put to bed and given salicylates for 6 weeks and kept away from school for 3 months.

Four days before he was admitted to hospital Tomas had again become feverish and listless and had complained of a vague pain in the upper part of his left arm and shoulder, later across the top of his chest. The next day the doctor heard a pericardial friction rub. He thought this was the result of rheumatic fever and sent Tomas to hospital. On examination Tomas was thin, wanting to lie still, but not unduly ill or distressed. His temperature was 39°C, respiration rate 24 and pulse 120. There was a marked increase in cardiac dullness, particularly on the left side. There was a loud pericardial friction rub through which the heart sounds could be faintly heard. There was no heart murmur. The liver was not enlarged. The neck veins were not distended. In the chest there was some dullness and decreased air entry at the left base.

Diagnosis: Because of the erythema nodosum and the presence of a pericardial effusion in a boy who was not as ill as he would have been with rheumatic carditis, the doctor thought of the possibility of tuberculosis. So he began anti-tuberculosis chemotherapy and then went on with the investigations. The tuberculin test was strongly positive. The white blood cell count was 8000, haemoglobin 110%, both unlikely in acute rheumatism. The electrocardiogram was normal but the X-ray showed a large heart shadow consistent with a pericardial effusion (see Figure 2.8, page 30) and some pleural reaction at the left base. Nothing abnormal was seen in the lung fields.

Improvement had begun within 4 days of starting treatment. The boy's temperature subsided. Although the friction rub remained for 10 days, the heart sounds became louder and were normal. X-ray on the 10th day confirmed that the effusion was smaller, and it had disappeared in a third film taken after a month. But in the second and third X-rays there was

cont'd ▶

evidence of enlargement of the right hilar lymph nodes. X-rays taken 3 years later showed calcification in this area. The patient made a complete recovery.

Tomas's family were investigated. His parents were normal and his brother's tuberculin test was negative, but his maternal grandfather was found to have active pulmonary tuberculosis.

5 Lymph node tuberculosis

Lymph node tuberculosis in adults is similar to that in children, as described in Chapter 2 (page 45). But a few points are worth emphasising.

▶ In older adults, remember the possibility that enlarged nodes may be due to carcinoma spreading from a primary carcinoma in the draining area. Hard nodes behind the inner end of the clavicle are often linked with a lung cancer. In some countries this will become more and more common as the tobacco smoking habit spreads.

▶ In adults, as in children, there is usually no fever with tuberculous peripheral lymph nodes, although sometimes there is low fever. Occasionally we have seen very high fever in adults whose chest X-ray shows enlarged lymph nodes at the hilum and along the trachea. There may also be enlarged lymph nodes in the neck.

The prognosis is good as far as survival is concerned. But if there have been many discharging sinuses, these may result in much scarring.

The tuberculin test is usually positive, but may be negative if there is malnutrition.

6 Tuberculosis of bones and joints

The problems are similar in adults to those in children, as covered in Chapter 2 (page 50).

7 Renal and urinary tract tuberculosis

How it arises

Renal tuberculosis is due to spread in the blood from the primary infection. Disease usually develops late, 5–15 years after the first infection. It is rare in children.

The disease usually starts in the outer part of the kidney (cortex). As it spreads it destroys kidney tissue and forms a cavity. If inflammatory material obstructs the junction between the kidney and the ureter, the back pressure may lead to widespread destruction of the kidney. Infection may then spread to the ureter (which may become obstructed) and to the bladder (where ulcers may form). It may also spread to the prostate, seminal vesicles and epididymis, although tuberculosis of the genital system often develops without renal and urinary tract tuberculosis.

Clinical features

The following symptoms and signs may be seen:

▶ frequency of passing urine
▶ pain on passing urine
▶ pain in the loin; usually dull, sometimes acute (renal colic)
▶ blood in urine: if the disease is mainly in the kidney, with little bladder infection, blood in the urine may be the only symptom (remember that a renal tumour is another possible cause; bilharziasis [schistosomiasis] is a common cause in some countries)
▶ swelling of the epididymis
▶ pus in the urine; culture for non-tuberculous bacteria will be negative
▶ loin abscess in advanced cases.

Diagnosis

The flow chart in *Figure 4.2* may help you in making the diagnosis.

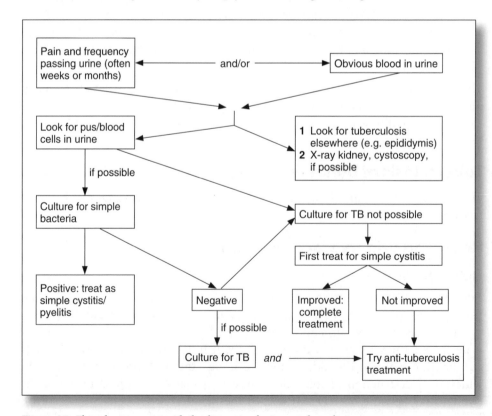

Figure 4.2 *Flow chart to assist with the diagnosis of urinary tuberculosis.*

Note the following points:

▶ *Urine*: Examine for pus and TB. Smear examination can be misleading. Harmless environmental acid-fast bacilli may be found in the urine. Don't rely on this for diagnosis unless over evidence points to tuberculosis. Culture for TB, if possible, is the reliable method but of course takes some weeks.

▶ *X-ray of kidney*: the best method is the intravenous pyelogram which can be very helpful if it is available.

▶ *Clinical examination of epididymis and testes* can be very useful. Examine the prostate by digital rectal examination. Instead of a smooth surface you may be able to feel craggy areas on one or both sides.

▶ *Chest X-ray*: usually there is no abnormality.

▶ *Blood urea* (if available) will tell you whether the other kidney is functioning normally.

If few investigations are possible and you cannot culture the urine or do X-rays, you will have to decide on clinical grounds whether to treat. Frequency and pain on passing urine will usually have come on gradually and will have been present for weeks or months before you see the patient. As acute cystitis usually starts suddenly, it soon brings the patient for help. Then look carefully for evidence of tuberculosis elsewhere, especially in the epididymis.

If in doubt, give standard treatment for simple cystitis. If the patient does not improve, you should consider that the patient has tuberculosis. Symptoms will usually start improving within 10 days after starting treatment for tuberculosis.

Management is described in Chapter 6.

A man with genitourinary tuberculosis

Mr Mwasa, aged 44 years, came to a health post in a rural area. He had had pain on passing urine for about 3 months. He had to pass urine frequently – he had to get up 5 or 6 times during the night. He thought that sometimes there might have been blood in his urine. He did not feel well and he thought he had lost weight.

The health assistant gave him a simple antibiotic for cystitis. After a week there was no improvement, so he referred the patient to the small district hospital half a day's walk away. The doctor there examined the patient carefully. He found an irregular, craggy, painless swelling in the upper part of the right epididymis. He did a rectal examination and felt an irregular swelling in the right lobe of the prostate.

The doctor sent the urine for examination. There were many pus cells and red cells in the deposit. Acid-fast bacilli were also present. There were no bilharzia eggs (bilharzia [schistosomiasis] was quite common in that area). On the basis of his findings in the epididymis and prostate, and the

cont'd ▶

patient's history, the doctor thought that this was a tuberculous cystitis, probably with renal disease. The acid-fast bacilli partly confirmed this. But the doctor knew that environmental acid-fast bacilli could be found in the urine, so that only partly confirmed the diagnosis. There were no facilities for culture or for intravenous pyelograms in this small hospital. The nearest hospital where this could be done was several days' journey away and the patient was unwilling to make the journey.

As the patient was not very ill and had a fairly short history, the doctor decided it was best to treat him with anti-tuberculosis chemotherapy and watch him carefully. But to be on the safe side he checked two further specimens for bilharzia eggs, both of which were negative.

Mr Mwasa's condition improved rapidly with anti-tuberculosis chemotherapy. His urinary symptoms disappeared in 2–3 weeks. His appetite increased and he gained weight. The doctor had carefully and kindly explained about the disease and the treatment. He had told the patient and his family how important it was to go on with the treatment for the full period, even if he might lose his symptoms and feel well after a few weeks. So Mr Mwasa came back regularly and finished his treatment.

Comment: Of course it would have been safer to have had an intravenous pyelogram and to check whether the ureter was obstructed, but this was not possible. The patient obviously did very well. Even if the kidney had been damaged by an obstruction of the ureter, usually only one kidney is diseased. The other kidney, if normal, could function normally and prevent renal failure.

4.8 Tuberculosis of the female genital tract

How it arises

Genital tuberculosis in women arises as a result of blood spread after primary infection. It affects the endometrium (uterus lining) and Fallopian tubes.

Clinical features

▶ Infertility is the most common reason for seeking help. The diagnosis is often made as a result of routine investigation for infertility. This should always include looking for signs of tuberculosis.

▶ Common symptoms include lower abdominal or pelvic pain, malaise and disturbance of the rhythm of menstruation (including amenorrhoea or unusual bleeding or spotting) or postmenopausal bleeding.

▶ It may progress to abscess formation of the Fallopian tube. Sometimes it is associated with large abdominal masses.

▶ Ectopic pregnancy (i.e. pregnancy in the Fallopian tube) may occur.

Investigations

▶ Pelvic examination may reveal masses, which may be small or large, over the Fallopian tube area.

▶ The genital tract should be X-rayed, if this is possible.

Treatment

Patients improve very well with chemotherapy. Large masses may just fade away. Surgery for these is unnecessary.

Although the disease is always arrested if chemotherapy is taken properly, damage to the Fallopian tube may obstruct its very small lumen and the patient may remain infertile. Because the ovum may not be able to get through the narrowed tube, ectopic pregnancy may occur later. Skilled surgical treatment of the blocked tube, if available, can sometimes restore fertility.

.9 Tuberculosis of the male genital tract

How it arises

The prostate, seminal vesicles and epididymis may be involved separately or together. Infection may come from the bloodstream or from the kidney via the urinary tract.

Clinical features

Most often the patient comes to the clinic complaining of something wrong with one of his 'testes' although in fact this is usually the epididymis, not the testis itself. The epididymis enlarges and becomes hard and craggy, usually starting at its upper pole. It is usually only slightly tender. An acute non-tuberculous epididymitis is usually very tender and painful. The lesion in the epididymis may break down into an abscess, involve the skin and result in a sinus. You should also examine the seminal vesicles via the rectum. The prostate may feel craggy and you may be able to feel the seminal vesicles on each side, above and lateral to the prostate. If you can feel them they are probably abnormal.

In 40% of cases the patient will also have the symptoms and signs of urinary tuberculosis.

Investigations

▶ Test the urine and sputum for evidence of tuberculosis.

▶ X-ray the kidney if this is possible.

▶ Tuberculin test is rarely helpful.

Diagnosis

▶ Acute epididymitis: fever, chills, acute pain locally.
▶ Tumour: usually smooth and hard. The craggy mass of tuberculosis is usually typical.

Treatment

Treatment with chemotherapy is normally completely successful if taken fully. Surgical treatment is only needed if a tumour is suspected.

4.10 Intestinal/peritoneal/abdominal tuberculosis

How it arises

Tuberculosis of the abdomen includes the abdominal lymphatic system, the peritoneum, the intestine (most frequently ileocaecal and anorectal), and the forms of intra-abdominal genitourinary tuberculosis discussed above. It is not always easy to disentangle these and be sure of the events that led to the presenting symptoms.

In some cases, the disease arises from blood-borne spread through the lymph nodes or the peritoneum. The lymph nodes enlarge and get matted together. If they rupture, infection spreads into the peritoneal cavity and effusion occurs (ascites); the adhesion of nodes to the bowel may cause obstruction. Communications (fistulae) may occur between the bowel and bladder, or between the bowel and the abdominal wall.

Patients with pulmonary tuberculosis may swallow their sputum. If the TB are abundant, they may infect the wall of the intestine (usually the ileum) or the area around the anus and cause ulceration, sinus or fistula. Fistulae may occur as described above. Infection may spread into the abdominal cavity and cause ascites.

Clinical features

There may be the following symptoms or signs:
▶ Loss of weight and loss of appetite are very common.
▶ The patient may have abdominal pain, which is often vague, fever, night sweats, or diarrhoea; menstruation may have stopped.
▶ Abdominal mass or masses may be found, often rather soft to feel. There is often also fluid in the abdomen (ascites) – sometimes there is so much fluid that you cannot feel any mass, so that the main sign is ascites. In hyperplastic ileo-caecal tuberculosis there may be pain and a mass to be felt in the right lower abdomen. There may be no signs elsewhere. This can be confused with cancer of the bowel.
▶ Attacks of intestinal obstruction with acute pain and distension of the abdomen may occur.

▶ Cough and sputum may be present if the bowel disease is caused by swallowing the sputum from pulmonary tuberculosis (secondary form).

▶ Ulceration, abscess, sinuses and fistulae in or around the anus in a patient with heavily smear-positive pulmonary tuberculosis is often due to tuberculosis and will respond to treatment of the pulmonary tuberculosis.

Diagnosis

Suspect the possibility of abdominal tuberculosis in any patient who is losing weight and who has fever and vague abdominal pain. Be even more suspicious if there is an abdominal mass or fluid in the abdomen. You will usually have to make the diagnosis on clinical grounds. But sometimes additional help may be obtained from:

▶ X-ray examination of the bowel
▶ biopsy of lymph node or peritoneum at operation or laparoscopy (examination via a lighted tube inserted into the abdomen through a small incision)
▶ culture of material from aspiration of liquid from the abdominal cavity or pus from sinuses.

Sometimes a patient has only recurrent vague abdominal pain. There may be no obvious fluid or masses to be felt. There may be little fever. If it is not possible to carry out any of the above investigations it is worth trying chemotherapy. If the disease is tuberculosis, the patient soon loses the symptoms and begins to improve.

Treatment

Chemotherapy is usually highly effective and even large masses fade away. Occasionally healed disease leaves adhesions between loops of intestine, or scarring. These sometimes later cause mechanical obstruction of the bowel and may need surgery. If there is a large amount of fluid you may have to aspirate it. It may be useful then to give prednisolone as well as chemotherapy, if available.

11 Tuberculosis of the eye

This may occur at any age. The different types have been described in the section on children's tuberculosis in Chapter 2 (page 57).

12 Adrenal tuberculosis

General comments

In countries where tuberculosis is common it may cause half the cases of adrenal insufficiency (Addison's disease). The TB reach the adrenal glands through the bloodstream.

The main symptoms are severe tiredness and general weakness. There is often recurrent vomiting and diarrhoea. A common and valuable clue to diagnosis is pigmentation of the skin, which occurs particularly over pressure areas (e.g. elbows or lower thoracic spine). It also occurs in patches inside the mouth: this is particularly valuable in races with naturally pigmented skin. The blood pressure is low. Sometimes the tuberculin test may be helpful.

The serum sodium concentration is often below normal, if you can test it, and is due to repeated vomiting and/or diarrhoea. High plasma potassium is even more frequent and is due to lack of aldosterone.

X-ray of the abdomen (if you can get it) shows calcification in the region of the adrenal glands in about 20% of cases. Tuberculous adrenal glands are usually enlarged, but this can only be shown by ultrasound or tomography, which is often not available.

AIDS may produce similar symptoms. Remember the possibility of Addison's disease, as you can treat this effectively. Remember to look for patches of pigment in the mouth.

Treatment

The tuberculosis can be cured with chemotherapy. Replacement of the missing hormones is always necessary. You must send the patient to an appropriate hospital specialist.

4.13 Cutaneous and subcutaneous tuberculosis

Cutaneous (skin) tuberculosis is not very common but the diagnosis is often missed. Correct diagnosis of the skin condition may help you to find tuberculosis elsewhere in the body.

There are a number of different types of skin conditions due to tuberculosis.

Primary lesions

See Chapter 2, page 60.

Erythema nodosum

This is a type of hypersensitivity to tuberculin. Usually, but not always, it occurs at the same time as the primary infection. It appears to be much rarer in patients with dark skin than in those with white skin, although this may be because the skin lesions are less obvious on dark skin. An Indian physician informs us that, after learning to recognize erythema nodosum in Europe, he has frequently diagnosed it in association with tuberculosis in India. Erythema nodosum is not only due to tuberculosis. Other causes include streptococcal infection, drugs, sarcoidosis, leprosy, histoplasmosis and coccidioidomycosis.

Erythema nodosum is rare before 7 years of age and is more common in females at all ages. There is often preliminary fever, which may be high in young women. Women may also have pain in the larger joints, which may be hot and tender as in rheumatic fever.

The most obvious finding is tender, dusky-red, slightly nodular lesions on the front of the legs below the knee. They feel deep to the skin rather than in it. They are 5–20 mm in diameter and have ill-defined margins. They may run together to become confluent, usually above the ankles. This produces a firm, tender, dusky-red area. Recurrent crops of lesions may occur over weeks.

If you suspect erythema nodosum, look carefully for evidence of tuberculosis, or one of the other causes given above. The tuberculin test is usually very strongly positive. There may be severe skin reaction to the normal dose of tuberculin, or even general reaction with fever. If there is tuberculosis, the erythema nodosum usually improves very rapidly with treatment.

Miliary lesions

These are rare but may become more common in patients with HIV infection and tuberculosis. They may or may not be associated with disseminated tuberculosis. There are three forms:

▶ multiple small copper-coloured spots
▶ multiple papules that break down in the middle and form pustules
▶ multiple subcutaneous abscesses on the arms and legs, the chest wall or the buttocks; perianal abscesses (abscesses near the anus) may also occur.

Verrucous tuberculosis

These lesions occur in patients with a good deal of immunity to tuberculosis. 'Warty' lesions appear on exposed parts of the body. Regional lymph nodes are not enlarged.

Ulcers of the mouth, nose and anus

These usually occur in people with advanced tuberculosis. They may be painful.

Scrofuloderma

This results from direct invasion and breakdown of the skin from an underlying tuberculous lesion, usually a lymph node, sometimes bone or epididymis. Sinuses usually develop and leave a scar when they heal.

Lupus vulgaris

This usually affects the head and neck. Commonly it occurs over the bridge of the nose and on to the cheeks. Jelly-like nodules appear and sometimes ulcerate. They may cause extensive scarring and destruction of the face. TB are rarely seen but the tuberculin test is usually positive. The condition is usually chronic and the diagnosis may be missed for many years.

Tuberculids

These are slightly painful, slightly raised, bluish-red, local, rounded thickenings of the skin. They appear mainly on the back of the calf. The tuberculin test is almost always positive. Such lesions are not always caused by tuberculosis but if you can be sure that they are not due to tuberculosis, you will often not be able to find the true cause.

Treatment

All skin and subcutaneous lesions do very well with anti-tuberculosis chemotherapy.

Important note

In countries with high prevalence of tuberculosis, do remember the possibility of tuberculosis whenever you see a chronic painless skin condition. If you suspect the skin diagnosis, look for tuberculous lesions elsewhere in the patient.

Chapter 5
Tuberculosis, HIV infection and AIDS

The rapid increase of HIV infection in many parts of the world is causing great problems in the diagnosis, treatment and control of tuberculosis. In 2005, about 40 million people worldwide were infected with HIV, 63% of whom were in sub-Saharan Africa and 22% in Asia. About 13% of tuberculosis patients globally are co-infected with HIV but in Africa this proportion is about one-third.

The problem of HIV and tuberculosis in children is discussed in Section 2.5 (page 68).

Note: Much of this chapter is based, with permission, on the WHO booklet *TB/HIV: A Clinical Manual* (see Bibliography).

5.1 Background

HIV and AIDS

AIDS is the final stage of infection with HIV. This virus seems to have first appeared in the world as early as the late 1950s. HIV gradually destroys the body's defensive cells so that the body cannot defend itself against infection.

In countries with a high prevalence of tuberculosis, 30–60% of adults have been infected with TB. Most people's defences prevent the TB from causing disease; however, if their defences have been damaged by HIV, the TB may not be kept under control and may multiply and cause disease. In the same way, people with HIV infection, even if not yet ill, may not be able to resist new infection with TB from other patients with a positive sputum. So there are likely to be many more cases of tuberculosis in countries where HIV infection is increasing. In some sub-Saharan African countries 20–70% of patients with tuberculosis have been shown to be HIV-positive.

Spread of HIV

HIV can be spread in different ways:

▶ between man and woman by sexual intercourse
▶ from man to man by sexual intercourse
▶ through blood by:
  – transfusion with blood untested for HIV (in countries where many people are becoming infected with HIV, even screened blood can be dangerous as there may be virus in the blood before antibodies can be detected)
  – use of needles that have not been properly sterilized (this is common in injection drug users)

▶ congenital transmission from mother to child, and also by breastfeeding; about one-third of children born to HIV-infected mothers are also HIV-positive.

Apart from sexual activity or blood contamination, there is no person-to-person risk. It is not dangerous to care for patients who have AIDS or who are infected with HIV, as long as you are careful about needles and blood. However, health staff who are known to be HIV-positive, even if healthy, should not care for patients with tuberculosis as they have a greatly increased risk of developing disease if they become infected with TB.

Geographical spread

The frequency of HIV infection in the sexually active population is already 15–35% in some parts of sub-Saharan Africa but seems to have stabilized in most. The incidence is increasing in many parts of Asia, and is increasing rapidly in the Ukraine and the Russian Federation.

In North America and Europe, tuberculosis is not very frequent among HIV-infected patients. Nevertheless, there have been important outbreaks of tuberculosis among the HIV-infected, some with multidrug-resistant bacilli. In countries with a high prevalence of tuberculosis, tuberculosis develops very frequently in HIV-infected patients.

There is a long period, often several years, between infection with HIV and progression to AIDS. This period is shorter in children under 5 years of age and in patients over 40 years of age. During this 'incubation period' the patient may feel quite well (though he/she remains infectious). The development of tuberculosis is often the first sign that the person living with HIV has HIV infection. In about 50% of patients with HIV and tuberculosis there is no other evidence of HIV infection. The only way to make the diagnosis is to do a HIV test. There is evidence that tuberculosis in an HIV-infected patient may speed up the development of full clinical AIDS.

In sub-Saharan Africa and now in Asia, HIV is mostly commonly spread through heterosexual intercourse. In many parts of Asia, HIV infection is increasing most rapidly among injection drug users. Tuberculosis may complicate HIV in both sexes.

Antiretroviral drugs

At present there is no effective vaccine for HIV. The newer drugs, especially if given in combination, do delay the onset and progression of AIDS, and these drug combinations must be made available to all patients known to have HIV infection whose clinical condition warrants their use.

Diagnosis and testing

You are most likely to see the patient at the time of presenting with symptoms and signs of tuberculosis or other infection. But often the symptoms and signs are unusual (see below). You can only be certain whether there was underlying HIV infection by doing a blood test for HIV antibodies. You must always ask the patient's permission to do this test. Where an 'opt-out' policy has been instituted, you must provide the patient with a chance to decline being tested. You must also counsel the patient carefully and kindly *before* testing, explaining why the test is necessary and what the result (positive or negative) may mean (see Section 5.6, page 125). This also means you must counsel the patient carefully and kindly when you get the result, whether it is positive or negative (see Section 5.6).

The HIV antibody test is the only certain way of making the diagnosis but this may not be possible where you are working. In that case you will have to decide by considering all the clinical facts in the patient's case.

5.2 Effect of HIV on tuberculosis programmes

Disease prevalence

In countries with high prevalence of tuberculosis, HIV infection is the most important factor that makes a person liable to get clinical tuberculosis. Among people already infected with TB (estimated from being tuberculin positive), the lifetime risk of clinical tuberculosis is about 50% if they have been infected with HIV, compared with a 5–10% risk if they are HIV negative. The result is a great increase of tuberculosis cases where and when the HIV rate becomes high. This puts a major strain on services.

Sputum testing

Sputum positivity is less common in tuberculosis/HIV, largely because tuberculosis is so much more frequently extra-pulmonary. The symptoms of HIV and tuberculosis are often similar. The result can be that health workers may make a diagnosis of sputum-negative tuberculosis and give anti-tuberculosis treatment when the patient's symptoms are not due to tuberculosis. So there may be gross overuse of anti-tuberculosis drugs, which wastes resources without helping patients.

Drug reactions

Drug reactions are much more common in patients with tuberculosis/HIV, which may increase the default rate from treatment.

Separation of patients

Patients who are HIV-positive should not be placed in the same room as patients who definitely have tuberculosis, or who may prove to have tuberculosis, as they are very likely to develop tuberculosis if they become infected with TB.

HIV-positive staff

For the same reason HIV-positive staff must not look after tuberculosis patients.

Needles

Great care must be taken in using needles. For this reason, streptomycin is no longer used for new tuberculosis patients in many countries with high HIV prevalence. (For full precautions see Section 5.13, page 128.)

5.3 Clinical appearance of tuberculosis with HIV infection

The following are differences from the usual way tuberculosis appears in patients without HIV infection.

▶ Extra-pulmonary disease, especially in the lymph nodes, is more common. There is often general lymph node enlargement, which is rare in other forms of tuberculosis.

▶ Disseminated disease is common. TB may be isolated from blood culture (which rarely occurs in ordinary tuberculosis).

▶ In the early stages of HIV infection with pulmonary tuberculosis there is often little difference in the X-ray from the usual appearances. In the later stages there are often large mediastinal lymph node masses. There is often lower lobe disease. The shadow may be only in the lower lobe and not very extensive. Cavitation may be less frequent. Pleural and pericardial effusions are more common. The shadows in the lung may change rapidly.

▶ Tuberculosis may occur at unusual sites (e.g. tuberculomas of the brain, abscesses of the chest wall or elsewhere).

▶ Sputum smears may be negative despite considerable changes in the chest X-ray.

▶ The tuberculin test is often negative.

▶ Fever and weight loss are more common in HIV-positive than in HIV-negative tuberculosis. On the other hand, cough and blood spitting are less common.

In a patient with tuberculosis, suspect the possibility of accompanying HIV infection if there is:

▶ general lymph node enlargement (in the late stages of HIV infection the nodes may be tender and painful, as in acute infection)

▶ candida infection (painful white patches of fungus in the mouth)

▶ chronic diarrhoea for more than a month

▶ herpes zoster (shingles)

▶ Kaposi's sarcoma: look for small red vascular nodules on the skin, and particularly on the palate

▶ generalized itchy dermatitis

▶ chronic increasing or generalized herpes simplex

▶ burning feeling in the feet (due to neuropathy)

▶ persistent painful ulceration of the genitalia.

.4 Note on WHO case definitions

The WHO has published revised case definitions for HIV surveillance and clinical staging of HIV-related disease in adults and children, after a series of regional consultations with Member States in all WHO Regions in 2004 and 2005, and deliberation of a global consensus meeting in 2006. We refer here to its publication: *WHO case definitions for HIV surveillance and revised clinical staging and immunological classification of HIV-related disease in adults and children*, published in 2007.

The WHO recommends that national programmes review and standardize their HIV and AIDS case reporting and case definitions in the light of these revisions.

Summaries of these definitions are given in *Box 5.1* for HIV infection and in *Box 5.2* for advanced HIV infection (including AIDS).

Box 5.1 WHO definition of HIV infection

Adults and children 18 months or older

HIV infection is diagnosed based on:

positive HIV antibody testing (rapid or laboratory-based enzyme immunoassay). This is confirmed by a second HIV antibody test (rapid or laboratory-based enzyme immunoassay) relying on different antigens or of different operating characteristics;

and/or

positive virological test for HIV or its components (HIV-RNA or HIV-DNA or ultrasensitive HIV p24 antigen) confirmed by a second virological test obtained from a separate determination.

Children younger than 18 months

HIV infection is diagnosed based on:

positive virological test for HIV or its components (HIV-RNA or HIV-DNA or ultrasensitive HIV p24 antigen) confirmed by a second virological test obtained from a separate determination taken more than 4 weeks after birth.

Positive HIV antibody testing is not recommended for definitive or confirmatory diagnosis of HIV infection in children until 18 months of age.

> **Box 5.2 Criteria for diagnosis of advanced HIV (including AIDS) for reporting**
>
> **Clinical criteria for diagnosis of advanced HIV in adults and children with confirmed HIV infection:**
>
> presumptive or definitive diagnosis of any stage 3 or stage 4 condition
>
> *and/or*
>
> **Immunological criteria for diagnosing advanced HIV in adults and children five years of older with confirmed HIV infection:**
>
> CD4 count less than 350 per mm^3 of blood in an HIV-infected adult or child
>
> *and/or*
>
> **Immunological criteria for diagnosing advanced HIV in adults and children five years of older with confirmed HIV infection:**
>
> %CD4+ <30 among those younger than 12 months
> %CD4+ <25 among those aged 12–35 months
> %CD4+ <20 among those aged 36–59 months.

5.5 Non-tuberculosis complications of HIV infection

You need to know about these as:

▶ you may have to distinguish them from tuberculosis
▶ they may occur in a patient in addition to tuberculosis
▶ they may occur later on when your treatment has controlled the patient's tuberculosis.

Early HIV illness

Most patients remain well after infection for months or years. The HIV only shows itself when the patient develops a complication, notably tuberculosis. But a few patients may develop an illness when their serum becomes positive for HIV, usually 6 weeks to 3 months after infection. The illness is often like 'glandular fever' (infectious mononucleosis): fever, rash, joint pains and enlarged lymph nodes. In severe cases there may also be aseptic meningitis, encephalitis (brain inflammation), myelitis (spinal cord inflammation) or peripheral nerve inflammation. These usually clear up without specific treatment.

Kaposi's sarcoma

Diagnosis is easy if you find small red vascular nodules on the skin. These may be less obvious on dark skin – look particularly at the palate where they may be more obvious.

Lesions in the lung or pleura are more difficult to diagnose. They are more likely to be confused with tuberculosis. The patient usually has cough, fever and breathlessness. X-ray, if available, may show diffuse nodules and/or pleural effusion. The effusion is usually blood-stained. If there is any doubt, treat the treatable diagnosis (i.e. tuberculosis).

Pneumocystis jirovecii pneumonia (PJP)

This is less common in Africa than elsewhere. The patient usually has dry cough and increasing breathlessness. In tuberculosis he/she is more likely to have purulent or blood-stained sputum and chest pain. In PJP, the X-ray may be normal or show diffuse interstitial shadowing in both lungs. Definite diagnosis depends on finding the cysts in the sputum or bronchial lavage but you may not have facilities for this.

If a patient with well-treated and controlled tuberculosis becomes increasingly breathless, first check that there is no increasing pneumonia. Also check that he/she does not have cardiac failure, asthma or anaemia. If you find none of these, the explanation may well be PJP. If you cannot test for this, try giving high-dose co-trimoxazole (3 or 4 tablets four times daily) together with a tapering course of prednisolone (if available).

Pulmonary cryptococcosis

This may look like tuberculosis. Definite diagnosis depends on finding fungal spores in the sputum.

Nocardiasis

This may look very like tuberculosis on the X-ray, and the organism may stain weakly acid-fast. Abscesses in brain or soft tissue should make you think of this possibility. Definite diagnosis depends on finding beaded and branching Gram-positive rods in a sputum smear. But of course look for TB first!

.6 HIV testing and counselling

HIV testing

A positive HIV serum test is proof of the diagnosis. If the test is available, consider offering it to your tuberculosis patients. Many will know that HIV is often associated with tuberculosis. Testing may have the following advantages for the patient:

▶ a definite negative test will relieve the patient's anxiety but counsel the patient about future risks and their avoidance (reducing the number of sexual partners; using condoms)

▶ provision of antiretroviral therapy
▶ better diagnosis and management of other HIV-related illnesses
▶ avoidance of drugs with a high risk of potentially fatal adverse effects.

If the test is positive, the patient must understand the importance of *always* using a condom during sexual intercourse, to avoid infecting others.

Laboratory testing

The standard tests are the rapid or laboratory-based enzyme immunoassays. If the test is positive, it is recommended that it repeated for confirmation. If the second test is negative, do two more tests to be sure the positive was not an error. In poorer countries it may only be possible to do one test and find it either negative or positive.

Pre-test counselling (see also Chapter 2)

Only test *after* counselling the patient on the advantages. Find out what he/she knows about HIV. Make sure he/she understands what a positive test would mean for his/her life. This covers both health and social/family aspects. There is probably a standard outline designed for the culture of the area where you work. There are probably local health workers, social workers or volunteers trained to counsel.

Post-test counselling

Counselling and support is obviously vital if the HIV test proves positive. Make sure the patient knows that tuberculosis can be cured in spite of the HIV. Work with any local organization for the counselling and support of HIV patients. Make sure the following are discussed:

▶ general health: diet, rest, exercise, avoiding infections (especially sexually transmitted infections)
▶ when to seek help for symptoms of other HIV-related illnesses
▶ possible side-effects of anti-tuberculosis drugs
▶ safe sexual behaviour with partners (reduce the number of sexual partners; use condoms)
▶ not to donate blood or organs
▶ patient's reaction to test result
▶ emotional and psychological support
▶ how to tell family, friends, lovers
▶ counselling partners
▶ social implications (e.g. employment, life insurance)
▶ referral to local support services and groups when available.

.7 Treatment of tuberculosis in HIV-positive patients

Short-course treatment

Modern short-course treatment of tuberculosis is just as effective in HIV-positive patients as in HIV-negative patients. The sputum becomes negative just as quickly but relapse rates are somewhat higher. Weight gain may be somewhat less than in HIV-negative patients. But with former long-term 'standard' treatment, not including rifampicin, treatment was less successful and relapse much more frequent. Some of the relapse may have been due to re-infection because of the patient's lowered defences due to the HIV.

Risk of death

The risk of dying is still higher in HIV-infected patients. Much of this is due to other complications of HIV infection (see below) but some deaths seem directly due to tuberculosis.

Prognosis

The long-term prognosis is therefore poor, as in all HIV-positive patients. But treatment of the patient's tuberculosis and antiretroviral drugs for HIV gives the patient a longer period of improved health. Moreover, anti-tuberculosis treatment stops the spread of tuberculosis to others. Unfortunately, tuberculosis seems to speed up the progress of the HIV illness. In addition to anti-tuberculosis treatment, antiretroviral treatment must thus be offered to all tuberculosis patients known to have HIV infection.

Side-effects

Side-effects of drugs are more common in HIV-positive patients. Tell the patient to stop treatment if he or she gets itching, and to report at once. This can prevent a severe reaction. If a patient develops a severe skin reaction to any of the drugs, never use that drug again. (Details of management are given in Chapter 6.)

Streptomycin

Streptomycin has to be given by injection, which carries a risk of spreading HIV from blood contamination in countries that cannot afford a new syringe for each patient. Thus, in countries with a high prevalence of HIV it is better to avoid this practice and to use ethambutol instead of streptomycin.

5.8 Treatment of HIV infection

Newer drugs given to HIV-infected patients do delay the onset and progress of AIDS. They are most effective if given in combination. While at present the drugs are still very expensive for a national programme in poorer countries, they must be made available to all patients known to be HIV infected. It must be made very clear, however, that even the best drugs do not *cure* HIV.

Your patients with tuberculosis and HIV may develop other infections and complications. For more details see the Bibliography (page 171).

5.9 Treatment of other complications of HIV infection

The WHO book detailed on page 119 gives details of diagnosis and treatment of other complications of HIV infection.

5.10 Preventive treatment with isoniazid

This is used in HIV patients with no evidence of clinical tuberculosis. It presents a number of problems: see Appendix C (page 164).

5.11 BCG vaccination

See Chapter 2 (page 72).

5.12 Conclusions

▶ With modern short-course treatment tuberculosis can be cured in patients who are HIV-positive.
▶ Giving good treatment to patients with TB and HIV prevents the spread of TB. This is particularly important when there are many HIV-positive people, as they have poor defences against the disease.
▶ Unfortunately tuberculosis speeds up the progress of HIV disease. Therefore your tuberculosis/HIV patients may develop other common complications of HIV. We have briefly outlined some of these. We have also listed some of the recommended treatments for them. For further details see the Bibliography (page 171).

5.13 Protection of health staff from infection by HIV

▶ Wear gloves when taking blood. Afterwards put the needle and syringe into a special 'sharp box'. Put gloves and swabs into a leakproof plastic bag.
▶ Wear gloves and an apron when doing anything that will bring you in contact with blood (e.g. surgery or delivering a baby). Protect your eyes with glasses.
▶ If blood or another bodily fluid is spilled, clean up as soon as possible. Use an antiseptic such as phenol or sodium hypochlorite.
▶ Use a bag and mask when doing resuscitation. Don't do mouth-to-mouth breathing.

Chapter 6
Treatment of tuberculosis

.1 General guide to treatment

Introduction

If the doctor prescribes the right medicines, and if the patient takes the medicines as prescribed for a sufficiently long period, all patients should be cured. The only exception to this rule is if the patient's TB are resistant to the drugs when treatment starts.

The aims of the treatment are:

▶ to cure patients with minimal interruption of usual life patterns
▶ to prevent death of seriously ill patients
▶ to prevent extensive damage to the lungs
▶ to avoid recurrence of the disease
▶ to prevent the emergence of resistant TB (acquired resistance)
▶ to protect the family and community of the patient from infection.

We describe below the medications that are used in treatment, the regimens (the frequency and combinations of the medications) and the duration of treatment. Before this we will discuss some general points about treatment.

Treatment is long, costly and somewhat complicated, unlike that for many other illnesses. Thus, treatment of tuberculosis must be a 'team' effort. This is important because every patient deserves to benefit from the special provisions for the treatment of tuberculosis (such as free medications) and must be supported to assure successful treatment. Before embarking on treatment of a patient with tuberculosis, it is essential to make contact with health services personnel from the National Tuberculosis Programme and to plan the treatment together with them.

A key point in the treatment of tuberculosis is that, when rifampicin is administered, every dose must be observed to be swallowed. This is complicated for both the patient and the health service provider. In addition, should the patient fail to return for regular scheduled follow-up visits, someone must search for the patient, even visiting his/her home. You must therefore think carefully whether you, as a physician, are prepared to do this and to do it conscientiously. If not, you must arrange to have this done by personnel in a clinic where the National Tuberculosis Programme is operating. Even if you choose to take advantage of this service, you will not 'lose' your patient, as you will continue to follow up the patient periodically in your own clinic.

When to treat (criteria for treatment)

Treatment is costly to the patient and to the health service. The medications used can sometimes cause harm to patients. Therefore, you should only treat a patient who almost certainly has tuberculosis.

Who should you treat? Clearly patients who are positive on sputum smear examination have top priority. You should also, of course, treat any patient who is found to be positive on culture and any other patient, including children, judged to have active disease.

The severely ill patient

If the patient is severely ill and sputum smears are negative, start anti-tuberculosis treatment. Get a chest X-ray if possible. If pneumonia seems a possibility, add a simple antibiotic to treat this. Antibiotics could be stopped after 2 weeks of treatment if the patient greatly improves. Once a decision is made to treat the patient for tuberculosis, any change in the treatment prescription should be made only on the advice of a specialist, because tuberculosis patients may become clinically well after 1 month of anti-tuberculosis treatment. If the patient gets worse, seek another diagnosis.

The patient who is not severely ill

If the patient is not severely ill and sputum smears are negative, arrange for a chest X-ray if it is available. If the chest X-ray shows abnormal patches or is not available, you may give a course of non-tuberculous antibiotics but *never use a fluoroquinolone*. Review after 1–2 weeks and repeat sputum examination and chest X-ray if possible.

If the new sputum smears are positive, or the patient has become seriously ill in the meantime, consider that the illness is due to tuberculosis and start anti-tuberculosis treatment, unless there is a very good reason not to do so.

If the patient has improved, if the X-ray is improving and if the further sputum smears are negative, discharge the patient from care, but tell the patient to return if symptoms come back.

Extra-pulmonary tuberculosis

This may be suspected if you have followed the advice in Chapter 4. Swelling of lymph nodes, pain and swelling of joints, and signs of meningitis are some of the reasons that a patient seeks care.

Supporting the patient to complete treatment

Unfortunately, many patients do not persist with their treatment. They stop because the costs to themselves and their families are high and they are feeling better. They fail to come back for their drugs, or they move to another part of the country without having made arrangements to continue their treatment in that place.

> **Important note**
>
> Getting patients to take treatment regularly for long enough is vital.

Most patients can be cured of their disease but this works only if the patient is supported. This support should follow the rules for helping the patient not to default *(Table 6.1)*. ('Default' is stopping treatment too early and against medical

Table 6.1 Preventing default (patient stopping treatment too early)

1 Be kind, friendly and patient.

2 Explain the disease to the patient and their relatives. In doing this, remember there may be local beliefs about tuberculosis.

3 Explain the importance of full treatment to the patient and relatives.

4 Show the patient and relatives what kind of pills the patient will take and how to take them.

5 Tell the patient and relatives about possible reactions to the drugs. Tell the patient to come and see you if there is a reaction.

6 Give the patient a leaflet about tuberculosis and its treatment.

7 Tell the patient and relatives about your local arrangements for supervision of treatment, such as:
   ▶ admission to ward/hostel
   ▶ daily attendance at centre near the home for the first 2 months
   ▶ supervision by volunteer or responsible person in the village.

8 Carefully tell the patient, and give a card showing the date and place of their next attendance. If there is a local calendar, different from the international calendar, give the date in the local calendar. The patient will understand that better.

9 Check the patient's personal problems and concerns (e.g. job, marriage, 'what the neighbours will say'). Give the patient kind and friendly advice about any problem. Because such counselling often takes time, in some clinics it is found better to get a nurse or health assistant with a good and friendly personality to do the counselling.

10 When the patient comes back for a new supply of drugs, remember to check the number of pills left over. This will tell you whether the patient has taken all the doses. If the patient has not taken all the doses, ask in a sympathetic way why not. This will help you to give the patient the right advice about taking the full treatment.

advice; see below.) Having the patient come to the clinic to take medications is one of the ways to support the patient. This provides an opportunity for the health service provider to discuss with the patient and for the patient to share any difficulties with the treatment or follow-up. Consistently, when patients are interviewed concerning this apparently disruptive requirement, they express appreciation for the care and attention they receive (see below). The main reason for observing the patient to swallow the medications, however, is to make sure that the medication is taken correctly and that resistance to the medications does not emerge in the bacteria while the patient is being treated.

The international standard of care for tuberculosis patients (the 'norm' for good-quality care) is WHO 'Stop TB Strategy'. With this approach, patients are provided with close and supportive care, they never run out of medications and they are followed closely so that it is much easier for them to continue with the treatment. A part of this approach is that swallowing each dose of treatment is observed directly by a health professional or by someone designated and supervised by the health professional. The advantage of this method is that you can be sure that the patient gets every dose. If the patient does not attend an appointment, it is possible to immediately search for the patient and determine if there are any problems with the treatment.

In this way, any problem with treatment or other illness or social problem can be rapidly discovered and the patient can be helped to continue the treatment. (For the other elements of national control programme see Table 1.1, page 11.)

Management of patients who fail to attend (late patients)

It is very important that the patient does not interrupt treatment. If the treatment is stopped, the bacteria may start to multiply again. It is particularly important that the patient does not interrupt the first 2 months of intensive treatment. At this stage there will be many bacteria living in the body and they can start growing very quickly if the treatment is interrupted. Every effort must be made to find the patient who does not attend a scheduled appointment.

While the first 2 months are most important, even in the continuation phase of treatment, it is important to locate any patient who does not attend a scheduled appointment.

We therefore recommend that whenever a patient fails to attend a scheduled appointment, you start looking for the patient immediately after the missed appointment and ensure that you find the patient within 3 days.

Actions to get patients back:

▶ It is important to know the patient's correct address. The best way for this to be accomplished is for someone from the clinic to visit the home of the patient when the treatment is first started. This can be done by a specially trained 'home visitor'. If this is not possible, and the patient is illiterate, have the patient ask someone in the community to write the address (or

instructions as to how to find the residence) on a card. In order to find the patient easily some clinics ask the patient to give three addresses:
- the home address of the patient
- the address of a friend or relative who lives nearby
- the address of a shop or restaurant or teahouse where the patient is known and the staff know where the patient lives or can be found.

▶ If the patient has missed an appointment, the best approach is a home visit to locate the patient and find out the reason the patient was unable to attend. The home visitor acts as a 'late patient tracer'. A good, sympathetic, persuasive personality is important.

▶ Reminder by post is not effective. Delaying the tracing of a late patient will often result in the patient being lost and unable to be brought back to treatment.

Preventing default (stopping treatment too early)

There are many aspects of this problem. It is your responsibility as the care giver to make sure that all your patients take their full treatment. If they do not, the disease is likely to return. When you decide to treat a patient, take sufficient time to talk to the patient and explain everything in simple terms. Further in-depth explanations can be provided by a trained and sympathetic nurse or health assistant. The very best way to communicate with the patient is for another patient (one who is currently on treatment or has completed treatment and is cured) to speak with the patient and explain the effects of the disease and the course of treatment. If the patient can read, provide a leaflet that sets out the important details of treatment. (You may be able to get this from your National Tuberculosis Programme or a national tuberculosis association.) If the patient cannot read, someone in the family or village can be asked to help.

Explain what tuberculosis is and how it can be spread. Reassure the patient that the disease can be cured if all the advice is followed. Explain what will happen if the full treatment is not taken – the disease is likely to come back.

Show the kind of pills you expect the patient to take – and show them a second time to make sure the patient understands. Advise the patient how often the pills are to be taken. Explain that even though they will begin to feel better, the treatment must on no account be stopped until the course is finished. In modern treatment there is no need to keep changing drugs; this is bad medical practice and confuses the patient.

Explain that, very rarely, patients get a reaction to drugs, and point out that the main ones are the return of fever, itching of the skin, rash, difficulty with vision and, if injections are given, giddiness.

One very important reason why a patient may not return to the clinic is because of the cost. For patients who are working, it may not be possible to attend during working hours because of the risk of losing the job, in which case the family could starve. For those with heavy family responsibilities, such as the mother of the house, absence from the home may not be easy. This is particularly important if the clinic is distant, as in rural areas. Try to make arrangements to help the patient avoid treatment failure for these reasons. The best way to solve this problem is to arrange for the patient to receive the treatment at the facility closest to the workplace or home that provides such treatment free of charge from the National Tuberculosis Programme.

Try to get the help of the patient's relatives and friends. If the patient gives permission, explain to them the way in which the patient should take the medications. Advise them to keep encouraging the patient throughout treatment.

Advise the patient not to take any of the medicines for the treatment for tuberculosis that can be bought in the market or are provided by other 'doctors'. Taking any additional medicines might cause serious reactions; before taking any, the patient should discuss it with you. There is no need to spend money on vitamins, unless they are prescribed by you for a special purpose.

Where to arrange for treatment

Treatment should be given as near as possible to the home or work of the patient. Otherwise there are unnecessary costs, and many patients are already poor and cannot continue their treatment because they (and their families) cannot afford it.

If the patient does not get the treatment at your clinic, choose a clinic of the National Tuberculosis Programme that is as near as possible to the patient's home or work. It is useful to have the tuberculosis treatment centre at the same place where people come for other medical purposes (e.g. maternity or immunization clinics, health posts (see paragraph above)). Try not to keep patients waiting. If they have long waits they may not come back.

Choosing staff

Choose with care those of your staff who are to provide the tuberculosis treatment. Make sure that they treat patients with kindness and understanding. One of the main reasons why patients do not return during their treatment is because the staff in the clinic are unfriendly. Choose staff who are keen on their work and who will do the work carefully and with enthusiasm. Encourage them when they do well. If possible, one member of staff must undertake clerical duties (keeping of records, etc.) and one should act as tracer of late patients (finding the patients who have failed to return and persuading them to continue treatment).

Patients' personal problems

Personal problems may also cause the patient not to follow the treatment, for example, the risk of losing a job, and fear about what friends and neighbours will say when they know that the patient has tuberculosis. These need to be discussed sympathetically with the patients and they need to be encouraged to share them with the staff members so that everything possible can be done to help the patient solve the problems. For this purpose, if it is possible, it is a good idea for patients to meet other patients who are much further along in the treatment so that they can support one another and share their experiences.

Drug resistance

This is important because treatment will not succeed if the bacteria are resistant to the medications used. There are three types of resistance: resistant mutants, secondary (acquired) resistance and primary resistance.

Resistant mutants

In any population of TB there will be a small proportion of bacteria that are naturally resistant. Therefore, the larger the number of bacteria, the larger will be the number that are naturally resistant. This particularly occurs when the number of bacteria are so large that they can be seen directly under the microscope (smear-positive cases). If only one drug is given, the sensitive TB are destroyed but the resistant ones multiply. *Never give a single drug* (monotherapy).

Secondary (acquired) resistance

Acquired or secondary resistance is caused by incorrect treatment:

▶ a single medication being given
▶ when two medications have been given but the patient's bacilli were resistant to one of them
▶ the patient fails to take medications properly.

Primary resistance

Primary resistance occurs when the person is infected by someone who has bacteria with resistance to one or more drugs.

The original cause of almost all drug resistance that is clinically important is poor medical practice. That is why following the recommended treatment plans and observing the swallowing of every dose of rifampicin is so important.

Follow-up

Sputum tests are the most important tests in the follow-up of pulmonary tuberculosis. X-rays add very little, if anything, to the follow-up, are expensive and in most cases are unnecessary.

Make sure you persuade the patient to come back to the same clinic for every scheduled appointment so that the staff can do everything possible to assist the patient to continue the treatment for the full duration prescribed. This also provides an opportunity to remind the patient again how important it is to continue treatment even though they may be feeling better. And of course this is how the patient gets the treatment.

Sputum testing

Collect sputum from patients for smear examination. For new patients, test the sputum at the end of the 2nd and 5th months and at the end of treatment. If the sputum tests positive at the 2nd month there are three possible explanations.

▶ The patient did not take the treatment as directed. It may well be that the patient did not come for every dose. Look into that very carefully.

▶ There is a large population of bacteria so they are slower to disappear (e.g. a patient with extensive disease and a large population of TB).

▶ Some patients continue to cough up bacteria that can be seen under the microscope but they are already dead (killed by the treatment).

Drug resistance is much less likely if you have given the treatments now recommended.

If you are sure the patient has taken all the drugs, you should give a further month of the full intensive phase treatment.

Management of treatment 'failures' is described below (page 144).

Relapse after successful treatment is very rare. You do not need to follow up the patient after the treatment is completed. But instruct the patient to report back if any symptoms reappear that suggest the tuberculosis has returned.

Outpatient or hospital treatment?

It has been proven conclusively that treatment as an outpatient can be completely successful. Admitting the patient to hospital for treatment is only necessary if the patient is very ill or if there are complications during the course of treatment.

However, outpatient treatment means that extra attention, care and follow up are necessary to ensure that the treatment is successful.

It has been calculated that there will only be an important fall in the amount of disease in the community if 85% of patients are cured (i.e. are documented to become sputum negative). Figures close to this, or even better, have now been achieved by routine services in a number of developing countries using the DOTS type of national programme. This occurs when the patients are carefully followed and supported and treatment is given near to the patients' homes or workplaces. Occasionally, because of distance or severity of illness, patients may have to be admitted to hospital or hostel for some of the treatment. If so, don't assume that if drugs are handed to patients they will be swallowed. Make sure that staff see every dose actually being swallowed.

Isolation

Long experience has demonstrated that, once good treatment has been well established, isolation is much less important. This remains true where HIV infection and drug resistance are rare. There is no increased risk of infection for the family whether the patient is treated at home or in hospital. The greatest risk of infection is before treatment begins. But there are a few groups of patients who may need isolation:

▶ *short-term isolation:* teachers and others in contact with young children
▶ *isolation until smear negative:* where there is contact with people whose immune system is not functioning well, such as those receiving immunosuppressive drugs (e.g. anti-cancer drugs) or who have HIV infection.

Inpatients known to have tuberculosis should never share a room with other patients. This becomes even more important where HIV is common and anti-tuberculosis drug resistance, particularly multidrug-resistant tuberculosis, is recognized as a problem.

Where HIV infection is recognized to be established (and always in institutions where persons infected with HIV are likely to visit), great care must be taken to separate tuberculosis patients from persons with HIV. In such settings, tuberculosis patients as well as any patients who are likely to have tuberculosis (especially those with chest symptoms) should not be admitted to general health services, if at all possible, before you are certain that they do not have tuberculosis. If it is necessary, great care must be taken to ensure that they are completely isolated from all persons who are potentially infected with HIV, including other patients and hospital staff. An important general rule is to never mix tuberculosis patients or those suspected of having tuberculosis with persons likely to have HIV.

Where drug resistance is frequent, the protection provided by treatment may be lost as a result of resistance to the medications used. When this is the case, once again, great care must be taken whenever a tuberculosis patient or a patient with prolonged chest symptoms is put into an enclosed environment with other people for a long period (any institution such as hospital, prison or residential school). If the patient has disease caused by bacteria that are resistant to a number of the essential medications used, the infection may spread from this patient to others in the institution. In this case, it is best to avoid institutional settings; if this cannot be avoided, the patient must be isolated from others.

Infants whose mothers have tuberculosis may die if they are removed from breastfeeding. They should be given preventive treatment with isoniazid. So should infants in close contact with any sources of infection. You should instruct patients in hospital to cover their mouths when coughing, as the main way by which the bacilli are spread is through small droplets in the air that are produced when coughing, sneezing or even singing or talking. There is no risk of infection from books and personal possessions. If a smear-positive patient has been in a room, when he leaves it keep the room unoccupied and well-ventilated for 24 hours. Then clean it thoroughly.

Contact examination

This is discussed in Chapter 1 (page 17).

Work

Work will not harm any patient who is not ill and who has been established on treatment. It is a great mistake to make the breadwinner or family supporter stop work because of tuberculosis. The decision about admission to hospital depends on the severity of the illness, national policy for tuberculosis patients and the economic effects on the family. You must consider all of these.

Lifestyle

It is best that the patient avoids tobacco and alcohol. But the most important thing is to persist with treatment. So pay attention to the advice you give if you think it will make the patient fail to take treatment. There is no need to alter established sexual activity because of tuberculosis, provided the patient is well enough. However, as always in life, everyone must take every precaution against anything that would promote the risk of HIV infection. In areas where HIV is well established (even if only in high-risk groups), advise the patient to be tested for HIV. Counsel the patient on how to avoid risks of getting HIV infection by: delaying the onset of sexual activity in adolescence, limiting the number of sexual partners, and through the use of protective devices such as condoms. Do all that you can do to make information available on preventing HIV infection, and provide access to condoms.

Pregnancy

It is best to avoid becoming pregnant during treatment, but there is no need to be anxious if pregnancy does occur. Give pyridoxine (at a low dose of 5 mg per day) with isoniazid to avoid any small risk of damaging the infant's nervous system. The other drugs in the routine regimens recommended here are also safe. But certain medications should not be given. Do not give streptomycin (or the reserve drugs capreomycin, kanamycin or viomycin): all these may cause deafness in the infant. Do not give the reserve drugs ethionamide or prothionamide, which can cause abnormalities of development in the fetus.

Remember that rifampicin increases the metabolism of oestrogens and thus makes contraceptive pills less effective. Always inform women of child-bearing years age that this is the case and that, to prevent pregnancy, they must rely on other methods of contraception.

The newborn baby

Manage the newborn baby as follows.

▶ Do not separate the baby from the mother unless she is desperately ill.
▶ If the mother is sputum-smear negative and the baby is well, give the baby BCG immediately (if it has not already been given).
▶ If the mother was sputum-smear positive during pregnancy or still is at the time of delivery:

- If the baby is ill at birth and you suspect congenital tuberculosis (see page XX), give full anti-tuberculosis treatment.
- If the baby is well, prescribe isoniazid 5 mg/kg in a single dose daily for 6 months. If the infant remains healthy, stop isoniazid and give BCG. Do not vaccinate with BCG at the same time as isoniazid is being administered.

Breastfeeding is particularly important when environmental conditions are poor and is to be strongly encouraged even when the mother has tuberculosis. Breast milk is far the best nutrition for the child. It also protects against many other infections.

5.2 Treatment for newly diagnosed patients

The first important task to be undertaken before starting treatment for tuberculosis is to determine what type of tuberculosis the patient has. First of all, you must find out if the patient has ever previously taken medications for tuberculosis (for at least 1 month). If so, the patient is a 'retreatment' patient and must be treated differently. It is often quite difficult on the first interview with the patient to be certain whether or not the patient has received treatment in the past. It is important to ask this question a number of times and in different ways and to reassure the patient that treatment will be given in any case.

Second, you need to determine if the disease is only outside the lungs (in which case it is extra-pulmonary tuberculosis). If there is any lung tuberculosis, it should be considered (and treated as) pulmonary tuberculosis. In any case you must be sure to examine the sputum to see if it is positive (it can sometimes be positive even when there are no other signs of pulmonary tuberculosis).

These steps have already been discussed but are essential before you can decide on the correct treatment for the patient.

National Tuberculosis Programme

Always use the regimen that your National Tuberculosis Programme recommends for the type of patient that you are treating. The recommended regimens are always different for patients returning to treatment after relapse, default or for patients who have failed on the regimen for new patients. In some programmes the regimen may be different for sputum-smear-negative patients or for children. You may find your national regimen or regimens below.

When there is no National Tuberculosis Programme

In the very rare instance where there is no National Programme we recommend that you use one of the regimens included in the 3rd (2003) edition of the WHO's guidelines: *Treatment of Tuberculosis. Guidelines for National Programmes*. The outlines of the different recommended regimens are given in *Table 6.2*. You will see that different regimens are recommended according to the type of tuberculosis case.

Brief method for summarizing regimens

The following method is now generally accepted internationally. Each standard drug is indicated by a capital letter. They are as follows:

Isoniazid: H
Rifampicin: R
Pyrazinamide: Z
Ethambutol: E
Streptomycin: S

Table 6.2 Treatment regimens adapted from recommendations of the WHO and The Union		
	Tuberculosis treatment regimens*	
Tuberculosis patients	**Initial phase**	**Continuation phase (daily or 3 times weekly)**
New patients, never previously treated for as much as 1 month	2HRZE	4RH or 6HE (daily only)
Previously treated for as much as 1 month: – relapse – treatment after interruption – treatment failure	2HRZES / 1HRZE	5HRE or 5HREZ
Patients with multidrug-resistant tuberculosis	Specially designed standardized or individualized regimens	

*H = isoniazid; R = rifampicin; Z = pyrazinamide; E = ethambutol; S = streptomycin
The number indicates the number of months that the drug combination should be given for.

All medications prescribed for the treatment of tuberculosis must be of proven high quality. Surveys have indicated that medications provided in private pharmacies in many countries are frequently of inferior quality and seriously risk the possibility that the patient may develop drug resistance. The safest and wisest way to ensure use of high-quality medications is to offer those provided free of charge through the National Tuberculosis Programme, which ensures their quality.

Best practice advises that, when rifampicin is prescribed, it should always be prescribed in a fixed-dose combination tablet that includes isoniazid. This is another safeguard to minimize the risk of developing drug resistance.

Drugs are most frequently given daily. The number before the drug combination shows for how many months that combination is given. For example, 2HRZE indicates that these four drugs are given in a single dose daily for 2 months. Similarly, 4HR indicates that these two drugs are given in a single dose daily for 4 months; 6 EH indicates ethambutol plus isoniazid for 6 months. The two standard regimens are:

▶ 2HRZE / 4HR
▶ 2HRZE / 6EH

This indicates that the four drugs are given for the first 2 months (known as the 'initial' or 'intensive' phase) followed by the two drugs for another 4 or 6 months (known as the 'continuation phase'), making 6 or 8 months in total.

More infrequently drugs may be given together in a single dose 3 times a week (intermittent treatment). This is indicated by putting the number 3, lowered by half a space, after each drug. For instance, if the first of the above regimen is given three times weekly instead of daily in the continuation phase it is written:

▶ 2HRZE / 4H$_3$R$_3$

The second regimen is only ever given daily.

Reason for giving four drugs in the intensive phase

Combined treatment is so effective because for each drug there are a very small number of resistant 'mutant' TB. If the drug is given alone, these can survive and multiply to replace the sensitive TB that have been killed by the drug. But the mutants that are resistant to each drug are killed by the other drugs. Even if the patient has been infected by TB resistant to one of the drugs (primary resistance), the other drugs will kill those resistant bacilli.

The same regimen for all patients

We recommend the above regimens for both pulmonary and non-pulmonary tuberculosis in both adults and children. There are some modifications in tuberculous meningitis.

Sputum positive after 2 months' treatment

With these regimens, about 15% of smear-positive patients will still have positive smears after 2 months' treatment. If the 8-month regimen is used, continue the four-drug initial phase for a further month before switching to the continuation phase. This will reduce the risk of treatment failure and relapse. But make sure the patient is taking every dose of treatment.

Drug dosages

The following dosages *(Table 6.3)* have been agreed by international experts. They are approved by the WHO and The Union.

Table 6.3 Doses of drugs for children and adults		
Essential anti-tuberculosis drug (abbreviation)	**Daily dose mg/kg (range)**	**Intermittent dose (3 times per week) mg/kg (range)**
Ethambutol (E)*	20 (15–25)	30 (25–35)
Rifampicin (R)	10 (8–12)	10 (8–12)
Isoniazid (H)	5 (4–6)	10 (8–12)
Pyrazinamide (Z)	25 (20–30)	35 (30–40)
Streptomycin (S)	15 (12–18)	15 (12–18)

*The recommendations of the treatment guidelines of the WHO will be revised to reflect the above dosages in the next edition.

For details about individual drugs, see Appendix A (page 149).

Fixed-dose drug combinations

These are now widely available. The advantage is that the patient takes all the drugs in the combination together. However, the pills or capsules must be carefully manufactured to make sure that rifampicin is fully absorbed. Each batch should be tested for this. Be careful to use only drugs from a reliable manufacturer. The best way to ensure the highest quality of drugs is to have the patient obtain those offered free of charge through the National Tuberculosis Programme. These drugs are certain to have been tested for quality.

Treatment in special situations

Pregnant women

Absolutely avoid streptomycin, as it may cause deafness in the fetus. Ensure that all women of child-bearing age are questioned carefully about pregnancy. Do a pregnancy test before prescribing streptomycin.

Women taking the contraceptive pill

Rifampicin makes the contraceptive pill less effective. It is best if the woman uses another form of contraception while taking rifampicin.

Patients with severe liver disease
Avoid pyrazinamide. Use one of the following regimens:
▶ 2HRE / 7HR   or
▶ 2SHE / 10HE.

Patients with renal failure
Isoniazid, rifampicin and pyrazinamide are either eliminated almost entirely by the bile or get broken down into non-toxic compounds. You can give them in normal doses to patients with renal failure. In severe renal failure, give pyridoxine with isoniazid so as to prevent peripheral neuropathy. Streptomycin and ethambutol are excreted by the kidneys. If you can monitor renal function closely it may be possible to give streptomycin and ethambutol at lower doses. Avoid thioacetazone. It is excreted partially in the urine.

Watch out for adverse effects of drugs – a symptom-based approach

Side-effects are shown in *Table 6.4* and are discussed in detail in Appendix A (page 149).

Table 6.4 Symptom-based approach to side-effects of anti-tuberculosis drugs (adapted from the WHO)		
Side-effects	**Drug(s) probably responsible**	**Management – continue anti-tuberculosis drugs, check drug doses**
Minor		
Anorexia, nausea, abdominal pain	Pyrazinamide, rifampicin	Give drugs with small meals or last thing at night
Joint pains	Pyrazinamide	Give acetylsalicylic acid
Burning sensation in the feet	Isoniazid	Give pyridoxine 100 mg daily
Orange / red urine	Rifampicin	Reassurance; patients should be told when starting treatment that this commonly happens and is normal

cont'd ▶

Table 6.4 Continued		
Major		
Itching, skin rash	Thioacetazone, but also rifampicin, streptomycin, isoniazid, rifampicin	Stop drugs
Deafness (no wax on auroscopy)	Streptomycin	Stop streptomycin, use ethambutol
Dizziness (vertigo and nystagmus)	Streptomycin	Stop streptomycin, use ethambutol
Jaundice (other causes excluded), hepatitis	Isoniazid, pyrazinamide, rifampicin	Stop drugs
Confusion (suspect drug-induced acute liver failure if jaundice present)	Most drugs	Stop drugs Urgent liver function tests and prothrombin time
Visual impairment (other causes excluded)	Ethambutol	Stop ethambutol
Shock, purpura, acute renal failure	Rifampicin	Stop rifampicin

Treatment failure and relapse

For management of a patient whose treatment has failed, or who has relapsed, see Appendix A (page 149).

Stories about treatment

Mr Masra

When Mr Masra, a 30-year-old man, went to a health post in a rural area he had a cough and sputum and had felt ill for several months. Three sputum specimens were positive for TB. The health assistant put him on standard treatment with isoniazid, rifampicin, ethambutol and pyrazinamide but did not fully explain the treatment to Mr Masra or his family. Mr Masra came back 1 month later. He was feeling much better and had lost his symptoms. He was given another month's supply of drugs but then he disappeared.

cont'd ▶

Six months later he came back to the health post. He said that 2 months before his symptoms had come back. He was now much more ill. His sputum was again positive. He said that after his last attendance he had felt well and thought he was cured, so he did not come back.

Another health assistant saw Mr Masra this time. He explained the treatment in a careful and friendly way to both Mr Masra and his wife. He gave them a leaflet on treatment to take home. Because Mr Masra had previously been taking all the drugs together, the health assistant knew that the TB should not be resistant. He therefore put him back on the same treatment. He explained to Mr Masra that he would have to start from the beginning again and take the treatment without any interruption for a full 6 months. At each monthly attendance the health assistant saw Mr Masra and talked to him in a friendly careful way. As a result Mr Masra took his treatment equally carefully and was cured.

Comment: The first health assistant did not take enough trouble to explain all about the treatment to the patient and his family. When the patient failed to come back, the health assistant did not send anyone to find him. The second health assistant was quite right in deciding that the patient's TB should be sensitive to all the drugs. He was also quite right to put the patient back on the same treatment. But this time the health assistant took a lot of trouble to explain everything to the patient and continued to encourage the patient all the way through till he finished his treatment and was cured. Of course it would have been even better if the health assistant was able to arrange for someone to observe the patient taking every dose of his drugs.

Note: In most National Programmes a patient who has relapsed will be put on one of the standard retreatment regimens (see Table 6.2, page 140).

Mr Chowdhuri

Mr Chowdhuri, a 40-year-old man, came to a district hospital with cough and sputum and was feeling ill. He said that 2 years before he was told at a rural health post that he had tuberculosis. He had been given pills for 'several months' and felt better. He then stopped treatment. A few months after this his cough came back and he coughed up some blood. This time he went to a private doctor in the nearest town. The doctor gave him some injections. Mr Chowdhuri could only afford the injections for about a month. But his cough disappeared and he felt much better. Now in the last 2 months all his symptoms had come back.

The outpatient doctor sent two specimens of sputum to be examined for TB. Both were positive. The doctor thought that the first treatment had probably been with isoniazid and thioacetazone, as that had been the

cont'd ▶

standard health post treatment at the time. The treatment from the private doctor was probably streptomycin injections. He did not seem to have had any other drugs with the injections. (Of course, using one drug alone was very bad treatment.)

There seemed a possibility that Mr Chowdhuri's TB might be resistant to isoniazid and perhaps to streptomycin. The safest thing was to put him on the standard five-drug regimen for retreatment patients who might have resistant TB (Table 6.2, page 140). The doctor therefore gave Mr Chowdhuri streptomycin, rifampicin, isoniazid and pyrazinamide, with ethambutol as the fifth drug. Streptomycin was given in case his bacilli were still sensitive.

The doctor also took a lot of trouble to explain to Mr Chowdhuri and his wife how important it was to take the five drugs with great care for the first 2 months. A health assistant watched Mr Chowdhuri swallow the drugs at the time he gave him the streptomycin injection. As he lived close to the hospital, Mr Chowdhuri attended for each dose thereafter, to make sure it was taken as directed. The doctor also explained to Mr Chowdhuri that if he had any trouble with his vision (due to ethambutol) he should stop treatment and come to see him at once.

The doctor saw Mr Chowdhuri regularly. Each time he talked to him carefully and in a friendly manner. He made sure he knew all about the treatment and how important it was. Mr Chowdhuri soon felt better. He completed treatment and was cured.

6.3 Treatment of extra-pulmonary tuberculosis

All these conditions, with the exception of tuberculous meningitis, require the same treatment regimen as for new smear-positive cases of pulmonary tuberculosis.

Pleural effusion

Use the treatment recommended for new smear-positive pulmonary tuberculosis. All patients should have full treatment. If not treated, 25% of them will later develop tuberculosis in the lungs or elsewhere. Where pleural effusions are particularly large or there are significant systemic symptoms, prednisolone may speed up recovery.

Pericardial effusion

If you can add oral corticosteroids to the chemotherapy of acute pericardial effusions, it is much less likely that you will need to repeat needle aspirations of the fluid. Use the standard chemotherapy.

Spinal tuberculosis

Use the treatment recommended for new smear-positive pulmonary tuberculosis. Most patients are now treated ambulatory, without bed rest, throughout. Controlled trials have shown that the disease can always be stopped by chemotherapy. Surgery is indicated to prevent or treat complications, such as nerve compression or the risk of serious paralysis in the case of tuberculosis in the neck.

Tuberculous joints heal well with the treatment recommended for new smear-positive pulmonary tuberculosis. Surgical treatment is required only if there are complications.

Renal and urinary tract tuberculosis

Use the treatment recommended for new smear-positive pulmonary tuberculosis. If the ureter becomes obstructed, the whole kidney may be lost. Back-pressure from the obstruction may destroy the kidney. To avoid this you have to know what is happening to the ureter. You can only find this out if you have expert radiology and can get an intravenous pyelogram. If possible, refer the patient to a centre where this can be done. *Figure 6.1* is a guide to management.

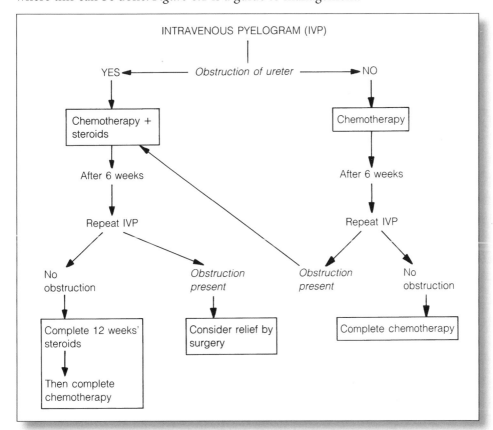

Figure 6.1 *Management of renal tuberculosis.*

If it is impossible to get a pyelogram, give standard chemotherapy for the standard time. This will stop the disease, but the patient may be left with some kidney damage.

Tuberculous meningitis

Tuberculous meningitis is the most life-threatening of all forms of tuberculosis. It is also the most likely to leave the patient with serious permanent damage. Therefore, the treatment should be as thorough as possible and should start as early as possible.

The treatment recommended is slightly different from that for new smear-positive pulmonary tuberculosis:

▶ isoniazid (5 mg/kg) with
▶ rifampicin (10 mg/kg)

initially with:

▶ pyrazinamide (25 mg/kg)
▶ streptomycin (15 mg/kg).

If the patient makes good progress, the intensive phase can be stopped after 2 months. Continue rifampicin and isoniazid for at least a further 7 months.

Oral corticosteroids (prednisolone) may be beneficial in cases of moderate-to-severe tuberculous meningitis to improve survival.

Where there is evidence of excessive cerebrospinal fluid pressure in the ventricles of the brain (hydrocephalus) or risk of loss of vision, surgery may be required. But this should only be done in a specialist centre.

Appendix A
Details of drug use

A.1 Drugs used in chemotherapy

This section gives details about the drugs used to treat tuberculosis. Use it for reference only.

The drugs commonly available for the treatment of tuberculosis are:

- isoniazid (H)
- rifampicin (R)
- pyrazinamide (Z)
- ethambutol (E)
- streptomycin (S)

Each of these is described in more detail below. The side-effects (toxic or adverse effects) of the drugs are summarized in Table 6.4 (pages 143–4).

Isoniazid

The advantages of isoniazid are that it is a very powerful bactericidal drug. It has very few side-effects. It is very cheap. Because it is so powerful, the dose is small.

It is normally given by mouth. Highly effective concentrations of the drug are obtained in all tissues and the cerebrospinal fluid. There is no cross-resistance with other drugs.

The rate of conversion to an inactive form (acetylation) varies in different races but is of no practical importance in standard treatment. However, slow inactivators are more likely to get the complication of tingling and numbness of the hands and feet (peripheral neuropathy; see below).

Preparation and dose
- Daily: 5 mg/kg up to a maximum of 300 mg in a single dose
- Intermittent (three times per week): 10 mg/kg

Adverse effects
Adverse effects of isoniazid are infrequent. Peripheral neuropathy (tingling and numbness of the hands and feet) is the main adverse effect. It is more frequent in malnourished patients and with high doses. It can be treated by giving 100–200 mg pyridoxine daily. It can be prevented by giving 10 mg pyridoxine daily. It is worth giving routine pyridoxine with high-dose isoniazid (for instance in three-times-weekly treatment):

- if there is much local malnutrition
- if the patient is getting many toxic effects
- if pyridoxine is available. (Your national programme may make recommendations about this.)

Isoniazid interacts with drugs given for epilepsy (anti-convulsants); doses of these drugs may need to be reduced during chemotherapy.

Rifampicin

Rifampicin is always given by the mouth in a single dose. There is no cross-resistance to other anti-tuberculosis drugs. Highly effective concentrations are obtained in all tissues and moderate levels in the cerebrospinal fluid.

Preparation and dose
▶ Daily or intermittent (three times weekly): 10 mg/kg to a maximum of 600 mg

If possible, it should be taken half an hour before breakfast. If nausea is a problem, it should be taken last thing at night.

It is supplied as capsules or tablets (syrup is also available) and should be given in combination with at least isoniazid.

You should warn all patients that rifampicin may colour the urine, sweat and tears orange–red.

Adverse reactions

Hepatitis occurring when rifampicin and isoniazid are given together is the most commonly encountered important adverse reaction to rifampicin. It is more frequent in older patients, in patients with HIV/AIDS and in those who are carriers of the hepatitis C virus.

The following patterns of adverse effects (syndromes) occur mostly in patients having intermittent treatment. They may also occur rarely in patients who have been prescribed daily treatment but take the drugs intermittently:

▶ 'influenza' syndrome, shiveriness, malaise, headache and bone pain
▶ thrombocytopenia and purpura: platelets fall to a very low level and haemorrhages may occur; it is essential to stop treatment immediately
▶ respiratory and shock syndrome: shortness of breath, wheeziness, fall in blood pressure, collapse; corticosteroids may be required
▶ acute haemolytic anaemia and renal failure.

Rifampicin should never be given again if the shock syndrome, acute haemolytic anaemia or acute renal failure have occurred.

Rifampicin and other drugs

Rifampicin stimulates liver enzymes, which may then break down other drugs more rapidly than normal. This includes the oestrogens in the contraceptive pill. You must advise women receiving rifampicin to use other forms of contraception. You may have to give higher doses of certain drugs if the patient is also receiving rifampicin. But remember to reduce the dose when the patient ceases to take rifampicin. These drugs include oral coumarin anticoagulants, oral diabetic drugs, digoxin, methadone, morphine, phenobarbital (phenobarbitone), dapsone, and, notably, certain classes of antiretroviral drugs (check current guidelines).

Urine test for rifampicin

Rifampicin can be identified in the urine by a simple test. Mix 10 ml of urine with 2 ml chloroform (analytical grade) by tilting gently in a screw-topped tube. The test is negative if no colour develops: a yellow-to-orange colour in the chloroform layer indicates the presence of rifampicin. The test will detect rifampicin for 6 hours after taking the drug, and up to 12 hours in some patients. Tetracyclines also give a yellow colour. A cruder test is just to look for the orange–red colour in the urine.

Pyrazinamide

Pyrazinamide is a highly effective bactericidal drug. It is particularly effective in killing off TB inside cells. It is very valuable in short-course treatment and in tuberculous meningitis.

Treatment and dosage

Adult dosage:

▶ daily: 25 mg/kg
▶ intermittent: 35 mg/kg (30–40 mg) three times weekly.

It is administered by mouth in a single dose. Each tablet contains 400 mg pyrazinamide (much preferred to the old standard of 500 mg tablets, which should not be used any more if at all possible).

Adverse effects

The most frequent adverse effects are liver damage (hepatotoxicity) and pain in the joints (arthralgia). Hepatotoxicity may be discovered only on carrying out routine biochemical tests. Anorexia, mild fever and tender enlargement of the liver and spleen may be followed by jaundice. If severe hepatitis occurs, do not give the drug again.

Arthralgia is quite common but is usually mild. The pain affects both large and small joints – shoulders, knees and fingers especially. The level of uric acid is increased and gout may occur. Simple treatment with acetylsalicyclic acid is often sufficient.

Ethambutol

Ethambutol is a bacteriostatic drug. It is mainly used to prevent the emergence of drug resistance to the main bactericidal drugs (isoniazid, rifampicin and streptomycin). It is given orally.

Preparation and dosage

Adult dosage

▶ daily: 20 mg/kg
▶ intermittent: 30 mg/kg three times weekly

Because of the risk of blindness, large doses are no longer given. You must make sure not to give more than the recommended dose.

Avoid in patients with renal failure.

Adverse reactions

The main and possibly very serious adverse reaction is progressive loss of vision caused by retrobulbar neuritis. When you start the patient on treatment, warn him or her about possible decrease in vision. The patient will notice failing eyesight even before anything shows in the eye when you examine it with the ophthalmoscope. If this occurs, the patient must stop the drug and report back to the treatment centre immediately, and there is every chance that their sight will recover. If the patient continues the treatment, he or she may become completely blind. Eye damage is much more common if the patient has renal failure.

Streptomycin

Streptomycin is not absorbed from the intestine so you have to give it by intramuscular injection. It diffuses readily into most body tissues. The concentrations are very low in normal cerebrospinal fluid but the levels are higher if there is meningitis. Streptomycin does however cross the placenta. As it is excreted almost entirely through the kidney, the dose has to be lowered in patients with poor renal function and in older age groups.

Providing syringes and staff to inject the drug adds to the cost and increases the danger of infection with blood-borne agents such as HIV if there is needle-stick injury or if needles are reused but are not sterilized properly.

Preparation and dosage

▶ Daily or intermittent: 15 mg/kg (maximum 1 g; reduce dose in elderly patients)

Streptomycin sulfate for intramuscular injection is supplied as a powder in vials. It is made into a solution by adding distilled water. Ideally, solutions should be prepared immediately before administration.

Make sure the nurse gives the injection into a different site each day. Daily injections into the same site are very painful. Because injection is painful, give streptomycin to children only if it is essential.

The nurse who gives the injections must wear gloves. Otherwise there is a risk of her developing skin reactions to the streptomycin.

HIV can be spread by infected needles. Whenever you cannot use a new needle for every single patient, or if you cannot be certain that sterilization is absolutely reliable, you should substitute ethambutol for streptomycin. This is particularly important if you are working in an area which has a high prevalence of HIV/AIDS. (But do not use ethambutol in young children as they may not tell you if they are losing vision.)

Adverse effects

The main adverse effects are cutaneous hypersensitivity and vestibule-cochlear toxicity (damage to eighth nerve). Streptomycin should be avoided, if at all possible, in pregnancy because it may cause deafness in the child.

Damage to the vestibular (balancing) apparatus is shown by giddiness. It may start suddenly and, if acute, there may also be vomiting. Unsteadiness is more marked in darkness. Examination of the eyes may show nystagmus (rapid eye movements). It is more likely to occur in older patients: attention to dosage is therefore very important. Treatment must be stopped immediately, if these adverse effects occur, as damage to the nerve may be permanent if the drug is not stopped when the symptoms start. If the drug is stopped immediately, symptoms usually clear over weeks. Deafness occurs extremely rarely.

Skin reactions – rash and fever – usually occur in the second and third weeks.

Streptomycin may be associated with an anaphylaxis reaction: the injection may be followed by tingling around the mouth, nausea and occasionally by sudden collapse.

Summary of adverse reactions

Isoniazid

▶ *Infrequent*: hepatitis, peripheral neuropathy, drug fever
▶ *Rare*: seizures, hallucinosis, psychosis, memory loss, optic neuropathy, pellagra, pyridoxine-responsive anaemia, metabolic acidosis, pyridoxine non-responsive psychosis, lupus erythematosus, haemolytic anaemia, agranulocytosis, pure red cell aplasia, alopecia, asthma, dermatitis

Rifampicin

▶ *Infrequent*: hepatitis, pruritis, influenza (flu) syndrome, drug fever
▶ *Rare*: interstitial nephritis, glomerulonephritis, renal failure, toxic epidermal necrolysis, oligomenorrhoea, amenorrhoea, anaphylactic shock, neutropenia, leukopenia, haemolytic anaemia, pseudomembranous colitis, eosinophilic colitis, lupus erythematosus, myopathy

Pyrazinamide

▶ *Common*: anorexia (loss of appetite)
▶ *Infrequent*: hepatitis, rash, nausea
▶ *Rare*: sideroblastic anaemia, lupus erythematosus, convulsions, photodermatitis

Ethambutol

▶ *Infrequent*: retrobulbar neuritis, periaxial ocular toxicity
▶ *Rare*: aplastic anaemia, eosinophilic pneumonia, thrombocytopenia, hyper-uricaemia

Streptomycin

▶ *Frequent*: vestibular toxicity
▶ *Common*: cochlear toxicity, hypersensitivity reactions
▶ *Infrequent*: renal damage
▶ *Rare*: neuromuscular blockade

Second-line drugs

These are active agents other than essential drugs and drug classes. These drugs are used for patients whose bacilli have been proved to be resistant to all the standard drugs. These are difficult to use and have many side-effects. They are less effective than the first-line drugs, and very expensive.

An experienced specialist must take responsibility for their administration, following the guidelines established by the National Tuberculosis Programme. The WHO recommends that the drugs should only be used in specialist centres. For guidance for these centres see WHO's publication: *Guidelines of the programmatic management of drug-resistant tuberculosis* (see Bibliography, page 171).

The following drugs are used as second-line drugs. The names are given here for reference only:

▶ aminoglycosides:
  – amikacin
  – kanamycin
▶ capreomycin
▶ cycloserine
▶ para-aminosalicylic acid
▶ fluoroquinolones
▶ other rifamycins
  – rifabutin
  – rifapentine
▶ thioamides
  – ethionamide
  – prothionamide.

A.3 Management of reactions to anti-tuberculosis drugs

These are important because they cause discomfort to patients and because they interrupt treatment.

Hypersensitivity (allergic) reactions

These rarely occur in the first week of treatment. They are most common in the second to fourth weeks. They are much less frequent with isoniazid, rifampicin and ethambutol than with streptomycin. Very rarely patients become allergic to all three drugs in a regimen.

There are various degrees of reaction:

▶ *Mild*: itching of the skin only; this is often the only sign of rifampicin allergy.

▶ *Moderate*: fever and rash. The rash is often mistaken for measles or scarlet fever. If severe, the skin looks blistered and the rash resembles urticaria.

▶ *Severe*: In addition to fever and rash there may be generalized swelling of lymph nodes, enlargement of the liver and spleen, swelling round the eyes and swelling of the mucous membranes of the mouth and lips. High fever, a generalized blistering rash and ulceration of the mucous membranes of the mouth, genitals and eyes (Stevens–Johnson syndrome) is a rare but dangerous reaction, particularly in patients with HIV infection. Very rarely chronic eczema involving the limbs may occur after the eighth week. This is almost always due to allergy to streptomycin.

Management
This is discussed in two parts: immediate and desensitization.

Immediate
▶ If the only complaint is mild itching, you can usually continue drug treatment, as the patient will become desensitized; you can give an anti-histamine drug (if available).

▶ If there is both fever and rash, stop all drugs; give an anti-histamine drug (if available).

▶ If there is a very severe reaction, stop all drugs.

▶ If the patient seems seriously ill, it may be necessary to send them to hospital for treatment with:
  – hydrocortisone 200 mg IV or IM, then
  – dexamethasone 4 mg IV or IM until the patient can swallow, then
  – prednisolone 15 mg three times a day orally, reducing the dose gradually every two days depending on the patient's response
  – IV fluids if required.

Desensitization
Desensitization should not be begun until the hypersensitivity reaction has disappeared. Management of desensitization is best done in hospital. It should NOT be tried if the patient has had a very severe reaction.

If possible, give two anti-tuberculosis drugs that the patient has not previously received while you are carrying out desensitization.

The challenge doses given in *Table A.1* are recommended for detecting cutaneous or generalized hypersensitivity to anti-tuberculosis drugs. Start giving test doses as shown in Table A.1. The reaction is usually a slight skin rash or slight fever and usually shows within 2–3 hours. You can therefore test two doses a day, at 12-hour intervals, if the patient is in a hospital or a hostel.

Sreptomycin is the most likely to produce an allergic reaction, so test it last.

Test all drugs the patient has received before starting desensitization because you may be able to give two of the drugs while desensitizing to the third.

Table A.1 Challenge doses for detecting cutaneous or generalized hypersensitivity to anti-tuberculosis drugs		
Drug	**Challenge doses**	
	Day 1	**Day 2**
Isoniazid	50 mg	300 mg
Rifampicin	75 mg	300 mg
Pyrazinamide	250 mg	1.0 g
Ethambutol	100 mg	500 mg
Streptomycin	125 mg	500 mg

From Girling DJ. Adverse effects of anti-tuberculosis drugs. *Drugs* 1982; 23: 56–74.

If you have other drugs available, it is often easier to substitute another drug for the one that has caused the reaction. If you do substitute a drug, check that this does not mean that you need to change from a short-course (6-month) regimen to treatment for 12 months. If you do not have alternative drugs, below is a guide to desensitization.

If a reaction occurs with the first challenge dose drug (as shown in Table A.1) you know the patient is hypersensitive to that drug. When starting to desensitize, it is usually safe to begin with a tenth of the normal dose. Then increase the dose by a tenth each day. If the patient has a mild reaction to a dose, give the same dose (instead of a higher dose) next day. If there is no reaction, go on increasing by a tenth each day. If the reaction is severe (which is unusual), go back to a lower dose and increase the dose more gradually.

If the patient is in hospital, or can attend at 12-hourly intervals, you can give the doses twice a day and save time. In most cases you can easily complete the desensitization within 7–10 days.

As soon as you have completed the desensitization to that drug, begin giving it regularly but make sure that it is combined with at least one other drug (to which the patient is not hypersensitive) in order to prevent drug resistance.

Hepatitis

All anti-tuberculosis drugs can cause damage to the liver, although this is very rare with ethambutol and cycloserine. It is very difficult to decide whether hepatitis is due to drugs or to infectious hepatitis in countries where this disease may be common. Hepatitis occurs as a side-effect in about 1% of treated patients, and is probably most common with pyrazinamide.

A mild symptomless increase in serum enzymes is a common occurrence but is not an indication to stop drugs. If there is loss of appetite, jaundice and liver enlargement, treatment should be stopped until liver function has returned to normal. Strangely enough in most patients the same drugs can be given again without return of hepatitis.

If the hepatitis has been severe, do not use pyrazinamide or rifampicin for retreatment. Give streptomycin, isoniazid and ethambutol for 2 months, followed by 10 months of isoniazid and ethambutol (2SHE/10HE).

If the patient is severely ill with tuberculosis and might die without chemotherapy, it is safest to give streptomycin and ethambutol (the least hepatotoxic drugs). When the hepatitis has settled, restart standard chemotherapy unless the hepatitis has been very severe. If hepatitis has been severe, use 2SHE/10HE as above.

.3 Corticosteroids in the management of tuberculosis

Corticosteroids suppress the inflammatory response to injury or infection. Consequently, they can occasionally help in treatment but may also be harmful. Never give corticosteroids to a patient with tuberculosis or suspected tuberculosis unless the patient is also taking effective anti-tuberculosis drugs. The only possible exception is the treatment of a severe allergic reaction to drugs.

Possible indications

Corticosteroids are definitely useful in the treatment of severe allergic reactions (hypersensitivity) to drugs, including patients with HIV infection and tuberculosis.

They are useful in reducing the out-pouring of fluid from serous surfaces – pleural effusion, pericardial effusion with much fluid and peritoneal effusion.

Corticosteroids help to reduce fibrosis and scar tissue such as in tuberculosis of the eye, the larynx and obstruction of the ureter in renal tuberculosis.

Their value in tuberculous meningitis has now been proved for certain types of cases.

Do not give corticosteroids routinely to patients with pulmonary tuberculosis. But if you have these drugs and the patient seems so ill that he/she seems likely to die within the first few days of chemotherapy, then corticosteroids may keep him/her alive until the drugs begin to work.

In disease of the adrenal glands (Addison's disease), you have to replace the missing adrenocorticotrophic hormones.

If you are not very experienced and do not know whether you should give corticosteroids or not, and if a senior colleague is available, ask for advice. Only give these drugs under medical supervision and in hospital.

Precautions

Remember that corticosteroids cause adverse effects such as fluid retention, moon-face, occasionally mental symptoms and worsening of a gastric or duodenal ulcer. In patients with tuberculosis, corticosteroids (such as prednisolone) are given for only a few weeks or at most a month or two. Therefore, long-term ill-effects (high blood pressure, diabetes, softening of the bones) should not occur.

Dosage

In mild conditions an initial dose of prednisolone of 10 mg twice daily for 4–6 weeks is usually enough. After that, reduce the daily dose by 5 mg each week.

In seriously ill patients, the dosage should be as follows:

▶ tuberculous meningitis: 30 mg twice daily for 4 weeks, then decrease gradually over several weeks according to progress
▶ tuberculous pericarditis: 30 mg twice daily for 4 weeks, 15 mg twice daily for the second 4 weeks, then decrease gradually over several weeks
▶ tuberculous pleural effusion: 20 mg twice daily for 2 weeks, and then decreasing rapidly. The dose for children is 1–3 mg/kg daily, divided into two equal doses. The higher dose would be for the more severely ill child.

In patients receiving rifampicin the dose of prednisolone should be increased by half for the first 2–4 weeks. The reason is that rifampicin antagonizes the action of prednisolone.

Steroids suppress the immune processes. So of course does HIV. But, on balance, patients with the above conditions are likely to benefit from the use of steroids even if they are infected with HIV, so do use them for these patients.

A.4 Management of patients whose response to chemotherapy is unsatisfactory

Defining unsatisfactory response

There are two situations that indicate unsatisfactory response.

▶ **Treatment failure:** the patient is supposed to be taking treatment but sputum smears remain, or become again, positive at 5 months or later during treatment.
▶ **Treatment relapse:** the patient has completed treatment and is documented to be sputum-smear negative but comes back to a clinic and is found to be sputum-smear positive again.

Investigations

When either treatment failure or relapse has happened, do not alter treatment without making certain investigations.

▶ Find out what treatment the patient has had – the drugs, the doses, the rhythm, the duration and whether it was supervised or not. If possible, get the information from the patient's clinic record card. It is a good idea to write the information down on a piece of paper – it often helps you to see the problem more clearly.

▶ Explain to the patient that the sputum test is positive (either remains positive or has again become positive). Speak to him/her kindly and say that to give him/her the best treatment now you must know what has happened: has he/she taken all the pills all the time? If not, did he/she miss taking them for days, weeks, or months at a time? If the patient claims to have taken all the pills all the time, try to interview a reliable member of the family (without the patient present). A relative is often more truthful, as naturally patients do not want it known that what has gone wrong could be their own fault. Of course, your proper attitude is that it is *your* fault for not fully motivating the patient and his family! Again, write down the result of your enquiries.

▶ Consider the possibility of HIV infection. Although most HIV-infected patients with tuberculosis do respond to treatment, they can become re-infected and develop tuberculosis again. Take a careful history and examine the patient for other signs of HIV infection. Counsel the patient and test for HIV antibodies if this test is available and if the patient agrees.

If you have a reliable reference laboratory you can send sputum specimens for culture and susceptibility testing. In most places this will not be possible, however. In any case it will take weeks to get the results and you have to decide how to manage the patient before you have these results available to you.

Treating the patient

The WHO recommends that all patients whose treatment fails or who return to treatment sputum-smear positive (whether after cure or after default from previous treatment) be put on a standard retreatment regimen (Table 6.2, page 140). In practice, most such patients do not have drug resistance.

Recommended retreatment regimens

The WHO recommends these regimens for patients who return to the health service sputum-smear positive after default, relapse or treatment failure. In practice many of these patients turn out not to have drug resistance.

EITHER:

▶ streptomycin plus isoniazid plus rifampicin plus pyrazinamide plus ethambutol, given daily in a single dose for 2 months
▶ streptomycin is then stopped and the other four drugs continued in a single daily dose for a further 1 month

▶ pyrazinamide is then stopped and the other three drugs continued in a single daily dose for a further 5 months, making 8 months in all
▶ summarized as: 2SHRZE / 1HRZE / 5HRE

OR

▶ the same regimen for the first 3 months
▶ followed by isoniazid, rifampicin, pyrazinamide and ethambutol for the last 6 months
▶ summarized as: 2SHRZE / 6HRZE.

This is often the patient's last chance of cure, unless second-line drugs are readily available for every patient in need. You must make sure that the patient is seen to swallow every dose.

Monitoring treatment

Examine the sputum for positivity at the end of the 3rd, 5th and 8th months (end of treatment).

If the sputum is still positive at 3 months, continue the four drugs for another month and then start the continuation phase. Make sure the patient is taking every dose.

Retest at 4 months: if the sputum is still positive get culture and susceptibility tests done if possible. But go ahead with the continuation phase.

If shown to have resistance to two or more of the drugs used in the continuation phase, refer to a specialist centre for multidrug-resistant patients. If there is no specialist centre, continue to the end of the retreatment regimen, making sure that the patient takes every dose.

If the sputum is still positive at 8 months (end of treatment), refer to a specialist centre if available.

Results

The above regimens should cure most patients who come for retreatment. It may fail in some of these patients, if there is already resistance to most of the drugs used (multidrug resistance). You should refer such patients to a specialist centre if available.

Identification of probable drug resistance through treatment failure

If a patient fails to improve and remains sputum-smear positive for 5–6 months, and you are quite sure that the patient has taken all drugs regularly, this suggests the possibility that the TB have been resistant right from the start of treatment. If the sputum becomes negative but later becomes positive again (and you are quite sure that the patient is taking all the drugs), this suggests that the TB may have been resistant to one or more of the drugs used to begin with and have now become resistant to the other drugs you are using, or the patient has been re-infected with a new resistant strain.

Unfortunately, this problem may be common in some countries. It usually arises because private doctors give short courses of a single drug (often rifampicin) or drugs in bad combinations. The doctor may have given, or added, a new drug each time the patient has relapsed.

If there is resistance to one or two standard drugs, the treatment given in Section A.4 should cure the patient.

If previous treatment suggests resistance to isoniazid, rifampicin and streptomycin, treatment is very difficult. The reserve drugs are weaker and have many side-effects. Refer the patient to a specialist centre. The specialist will start with four or five drugs, using drugs the patient has not had before, or drugs already used but to which the patient's bacilli are probably sensitive. When the sputum has become negative, one or two of the weaker or more toxic drugs will be stopped. Treatment will continue for at least 18 months. This treatment can be successful, but it needs skilful supervision and encouragement of the patient to tolerate the unpleasant side-effects of the drugs.

As such treatment is expensive, highly specialized and very difficult, national control programmes have developed highly specialized centres (perhaps more than one in big countries) where such patients may be treated (part of the WHO's 'Stop TB' Strategy). The WHO has produced special guidelines, for use only by such specialist centres (see the Bibliography, page 171).

Appendix B
Surgery in tuberculosis

Chemotherapy is always the most important treatment for tuberculosis. The role of surgery is almost always in the management of complications of the disease. It should be undertaken only in well-equipped and well-staffed centres. The indications for surgery are listed below. You should be able to cure almost all your tuberculosis patients without surgery.

B.1 Pleuropulmonary disease

Selected patients with drug-resistant TB who have failed on retreatment with reserve drugs may require resection of lung. In most of these patients lung destruction will be too extensive and the patient will not be suitable for surgery. In any case, surgery is highly dangerous unless there are at least two reserve drugs to cover the operation and the postoperative period.

Surgery may be appropriate for patients whose tuberculosis had been cured but nevertheless have recurrent severe haemoptysis from an open cavity or bronchiectasis. This may follow infection of an open cavity with the fungus *Aspergillus fumigatus*.

Very rarely, children or young adults may require surgical removal of mediastinal glands that are pressing on the trachea or large bronchi – sometimes as an emergency.

A tuberculous empyema that has failed to clear may require surgical removal.

If there is a round solid (coin) lesion in the lung there is sometimes doubt as to whether it is a tuberculoma or a tumour. It is thus best to remove it.

B.2 Lymph node disease

Surgical removal of lymph nodes is almost never needed nowadays. Occasionally it is used for diagnosis if the cause of the lymph node enlargement is very difficult to determine. If a lymph node biopsy is performed, it is best to submit the biopsy for culture for *Mycobacterium tuberculosis* or, at the very least, for histological examination.

Surgery has no role whatsoever in the treatment of tuberculous lymphadenitis. When the complication of a large lymph node abscess requires intervention, it is best to remove its contents rather than to aspirate it by needle.

B.3 Bone and joint disease

Surgical treatment is indicated to treat complications of spinal tuberculosis. It is indicated for decompression when collapse of vertebrae and collections of caseous material produce or threaten paralysis of limbs.

Tuberculosis of joints rarely requires surgery except for reconstruction of deformities following cure with chemotherapy.

.4 Genitourinary disease

Surgery is only indicated for complications but never for primary treatment of tuberculosis, which is accomplished by chemotherapy.

.5 Abdominal tuberculosis

This form of the disease responds very well to chemotherapy. The abdominal contents are usually so matted together that any operation is very difficult and risky. Surgery is sometimes necessary to relieve intestinal obstruction caused by residual adhesions.

.6 Tuberculosis of the thyroid or breast

Surgical removal of a mass may be carried out because the diagnosis is in doubt, and you suspect a possible cancer.

.7 Tuberculosis of the pericardium

Open drainage is seldom necessary in the acute stage.

Removal of a thickened and partly calcified pericardium may be needed if, in the process of healing, the disease causes constriction of the heart and interferes with its proper action.

Appendix C
Prophylactic treatment and preventive therapy

Preventive therapy has always been recommended for specific groups in every country (including developing countries): this group includes small children with household contact with sputum-smear-positive patients. This has rarely been put into practice systematically, although this is now beginning to change. In addition, other high-risk groups (persons with HIV/AIDS) are included in these recommendations. But you should follow the recommendations of your National Tuberculosis Programme.

Two terms are used to describe the two different types of preventive therapy:

▶ **prophylactic treatment (primary prophylaxis):** a drug is given to individuals who have not been infected, in order to prevent development of disease (e.g. infants being breastfed; whole communities)

▶ **preventive therapy (secondary prophylaxis):** the drug is used to prevent development of the disease in people who have already been infected with TB.

C.1 Drugs

Isoniazid is usually used for preventive therapy – it is cheap, has very few side-effects, it can be taken by mouth, and it has been proved to be effective.

The dose of isoniazid to be used is 5 mg/kg (not exceeding 300 mg) orally every day for a minimum of 6 months, but preferably for 9–12 months.

C.2 Use

If you are considering either preventive therapy or prophylactic treatment, remember that it is difficult enough to persuade people with tuberculosis to take treatment for a long time. How much more difficult will it be to persuade people who are well to take daily medicine for months, or give it to their children? The following are possible reasons for the use of preventive or prophylactic therapy with isoniazid. In some of these you may not know whether or not the person has already been infected with TB. But the treatment is the same:

▶ patients infected with HIV or who have AIDS
▶ breastfeeding infants of sputum-positive mothers
▶ household contacts of smear-positive patients, aged 5 years or under, who are apparently healthy – an age group liable to tuberculous meningitis or miliary tuberculosis (your National Programme may provide guidance for children older than 5)
▶ newly infected patients as shown by recent change in tuberculin test from negative to positive

▶ certain clinical states in which tuberculosis is more likely to develop (e.g. patients who have received solid organ transplants, those taking anti-cancer drugs and those with severe diabetes mellitus).

C.3 Doubtfully active tuberculosis

If you have a patient with a chest X-ray showing what seems to be a doubtfully active tuberculous condition or a patient with a clinical indication (chest or other suggestive symptoms) *do not* give prophylactic treatment with isoniazid.

Before considering preventive therapy, be certain that the patient does not have active tuberculosis, particularly if the person has HIV/AIDS.

Appendix D
Infections with environmental mycobacteria

These are sometimes called 'atypical', 'opportunistic' or 'mycobacteria other than tubercle bacilli'. There are a number of different sorts of these bacteria. They are common in our environment, in the water and soil for example, and some cause tuberculosis-like disease in various animals. They occasionally infect people and cause chest disease that resembles tuberculosis. Diagnosis can only be made by culture.

Rarely, particularly in patients with AIDS, the bacteria spread through the bloodstream. They may then cause multiple bone abscesses etc.

In countries with a high prevalence of tuberculosis these infections are less frequent, while tuberculosis is common. They will therefore be less important in your practice. In any case, you need culture facilities to diagnose infection with these myobacteria. So we are only mentioning these infections briefly.

Most people easily control the infection and do not become ill. But patients with AIDS have severely damaged immune defences and are particularly prone to these infections.

These bacteria are often resistant to some of the usual drugs used for treating tuberculosis. Therefore only experienced specialists should treat these patients.

Appendix E
Tuberculin testing

Infection with TB leads to the development of allergy to the tuberculin protein. When tuberculin is injected into the skin of an infected person, a delayed local reaction (inflammatory swelling) develops in 24–48 hours. We list below conditions that may depress this reaction. The reaction measures the degree of allergy; it does not measure immunity. It does NOT indicate the presence or extent of disease.

A positive test shows only that the person has at some time been infected with TB. The proportion of people with positive tests will increase steadily with age. Many adults who are quite well will have positive tests.

Below we describe the material used in tuberculin testing and how to interpret the tests. Using a syringe and needle always carries a risk of spreading infection (HIV, hepatitis). Always use a separate syringe and needle for each person.

E.1 Tuberculin

Recommended tuberculin

Internationally the WHO and The Union recommend using only-tuberculin PPD. This is a purified tuberculin.

Storage

Keep tuberculin at a temperature not higher than 20°C, except for short periods when using it. Do not leave it in direct sunlight or strong daylight. Do not let it freeze. The best temperature for storage is 2–8°C. Do not keep opened vials of tuberculin for more than 2 days.

E.2 The Mantoux test

The intradermal test after Mantoux is now the only test recommended by the WHO and The Union.

This section is based on The Union recommendations (see Bibliography, page 171).

Dose

The standard dose for both diagnostic work and surveys is 5 tuberculin units (TU) of PPD-S. This tuberculin is used only to standardize commercially available tuberculins and is not available for the general public.

In 1958, the State Serum Institute in Denmark prepared a very large batch of tuberculin for UNICEF and the WHO. It is called PPD-RT23. It is mixed with

Tween 80 (a detergent to prevent the tuberculin sticking to the glass). Of this tuberculin, 2 TU in 0.1 ml gives the same result as 5 TU of PPD-S.

There are other commercially available tuberculins that might be used in your country. Use your country's tuberculin, if it is standardized to give the same result as the international standard of 5 TU tuberculin PPD-S.

Administration

Choose an area of skin at the junction of the mid and upper thirds of the dorsal surface of the forearm (its smoother surface makes testing easier). If you always choose the left arm, you will not be looking for the result on the wrong arm. Do not clean the arm with acetone or ether. If you use soap and water, be sure that the arm is dry before carrying out the test. In a struggling child, ask a nurse or a relative to hold the arm steady (gently but firmly).

Use the special disposable 1 ml syringe (graduated in 100ths of a millilitre) and a 26-gauge 10 mm long disposable needle with a short bevel. (You can use 25 gauge if you cannot get 26 gauge.) Use a separate sterile syringe and needle for each person tested.

Draw up a little more than 0.1 ml into the syringe. Hold the syringe up and expel any air. Then adjust to exactly 0.1 ml by expelling extra solution.

Lightly stretch the skin. Insert the needle with the bevel upmost *into* (not under) the skin. Do not touch the plunger until the needle point is in the right place. Inject the exact volume of 0.1 ml. Remove your finger from the plunger before you withdraw the needle. This should produce a flat, pale bump (weal) with well-marked pits and a steep borderline.

If there is significant leakage of tuberculin (at the connection of needle and syringe or because the needle was not right in the skin), repeat the test more correctly on the other arm; make a special note of which arm has the good test so that you read the test on the correct arm.

Reading and interpreting the result

Read the test after 48–72 hours. If a reaction has taken place you will see an area of erythema (redness) –which may be difficult to see on dark skin – and an area of induration (thickening) of the skin. You can feel the thickening even if you cannot see it (try this with your eyes closed). Measure the diameter of induration across the transverse axis of the arm *(Figure A.1)*. It is easiest to do this by feeling the edges of the swelling and marking them with a ballpoint pen. You can then measure the distance between the two marks with a transparent ruler. Record this diameter carefully and precisely ('Mantoux 12 mm').

The amount of erythema (redness) present is not important.

The definition of a 'positive' or a 'negative' test is not the same in every place. You should use the recommendation in your country. Remember that malnutrition or severe illness, among other things, can make the test negative.

Mantoux tuberculin test

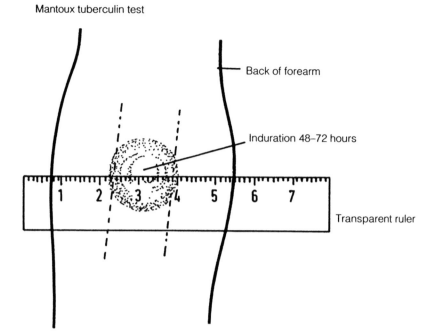

Back of forearm

Induration 48–72 hours

Transparent ruler

RECORDING THE TEST
1. Dose of tuberculin used (IU)
2. Time from test to reading it
3. Diameter of **induration** (not redness) in mm

Figure A.1 *The Mantoux tuberculin test.* Record the horizontal width in mm of induration (the thickening of the skin, not the redness).

For a particular patient you will have to consider the result of the test together with all the other information about that patient.

The more positive the test, the more important it is as evidence that you may be dealing with a person who has been infected with TB. But remember that it indicates only the presence of infection, which is one point in favour of the diagnosis of tuberculosis. Many well people have a strongly positive test. However, a strongly positive test is a particularly valuable point in a child, especially a very young child, as this indicates that the patient was infected relatively recently and is at a higher risk of developing tuberculosis.

On the other hand, a negative test does not exclude tuberculosis. A patient with active tuberculosis may have the tuberculin test suppressed by a number of factors such as malnutrition, viral infections, HIV infection, measles, chickenpox, glandular fever, cancer, severe bacteriological infections (including tuberculosis), corticosteroids and similar drugs.

A positive result is usual after previous BCG vaccination, at least for a number of years, but will become weaker over time.

Appendix F
Gastric aspiration in children

In adults the diagnosis of pulmonary tuberculosis depends on finding TB in the sputum. But children under the age of 5 years swallow their sputum and they are unlikely to be able to produce a specimen for examination.

When you cannot obtain sputum the only effective method is gastric aspiration. This method is distressing to the child, so only use it when you can culture the specimen for TB and when there is a particularly difficult clinical problem. If you do use it, pay particular attention to the following detail.

Two people are needed to perform the test.

It is best to get the specimen of stomach contents first thing in the morning, before the child has had anything to eat or drink. Children should preferably fast for 4 hours. Get your assistant to hold the child on the back or side. Attach the syringe to the catheter. Pass the catheter into the stomach. Check that the catheter is in the stomach by withdrawing 2–5 ml of fluid and testing it with litmus paper. Blue litmus paper turns red when brought into contact with acidic stomach content. Then suck the contents into a large syringe. The amount will vary from a few ml to about 50 ml. If the tube blocks while sucking, inject a few ml of water (5–10 ml). If that is necessary, wait a few minutes. Then suck again with the syringe. The ideal amount of fluid to collect is 5–10 ml. Place the material in a sterile container (sputum collection cup). Add an equal amount of 8% sodium bicarbonate solution. Close the collection cup and label the specimen. Transport the specimen in a cool box to the laboratory as soon as possible. If it is likely to take more than 4 hours to transport the specimen to the laboratory, place the specimen in a refrigerator (4–8°C).

In the laboratory the specimen can now be concentrated and a portion stained for TB. The rest of the specimen is used in the culture of TB. Microscopy can give you false-positive results, so culture is always indicated if possible.

Gastric aspiration should be performed on three consecutive mornings on each patient.

A positive culture of TB is obtained in fewer than half of children with pulmonary tuberculosis. If TB are not cultured from the gastric aspirate, this does not exclude tuberculosis. In this scenario you will have to use your clinical judgment to decide if the child has tuberculosis.

Bibliography

The following are useful publications and can be obtained from the addresses given on page 172.

Gie R. *Diagnostic Atlas of Intrathoracic Tuberculosis in Children.* Paris: International Union Against Tuberculosis and Lung Disease, 2003

Harries A, Maher D, Graham S, et al. *TB/HIV. A Clinical Manual,* 2nd edn. Geneva: WHO, 2004

International Union Against Tuberculosis and Lung Disease. *Management of the child with a cough or difficult breathing. A guide for low income countries.* Paris: International Union against Tuberculosis and Lung Disease, 2005

International Union Against Tuberculosis and Lung Disease. *Management of tuberculosis. A guide for the essentials of good practice,* 6th edn. Paris: International Union Against Tuberculosis and Lung Disease, 2009

Tuberculosis Coalition for Technical Assistance. *International standards for tuberculosis care (ISTC).* The Hague: Tuberculosis Coalition for Technical Assistance, 2006

World Health Organization. *Pocket book of hospital care of children. Guidelines for the management of common illnesses with limited resources.* Geneva: WHO, 2005

World Health Organization Global Programme on AIDS. *Counselling for HIV/AIDS: a key to caring.* Geneva: WHO, 1995

World Health Organization Global Programme on AIDS. *AIDS Homecare Handbook.* Geneva: WHO, 1993

World Health Organization Global Programme on AIDS. *Management of sexually transmitted diseases.* Geneva: WHO, 1991

World Health Organization. *WHO case definitions for HIV surveillance and revised clinical staging and immunological classification of HIV-related disease in adults and children.* Geneva: WHO, 2007

World Health Organization. *Treatment of tuberculosis: guidelines for national programmes,* 3rd edn. Geneva: WHO, 2003; document WHO/CDS/TB/2003.313:1–108

World Health Organization. *Guidelines for establishing DOTS-Plus projects for the managment of multidrug-resistant tuberculosis (MDR-TB).* Geneva: WHO 2000; Document WHO/CDS/TB/2000.279:1–87

World Health Organization. *Guidance for national tuberculosis programmes on the management of tuberculosis in children.* Geneva: WHO, 2006; document WHO/HTM/TBM/2006.371:1–41

World Health Organization. *Guidelines of the programmatic management of drug-resistant tuberculosis.* Geneva: WHO, 2006; document WHO/HTM/TB/2006.361:1–174

World Health Organization. *TB/HIV. A clinical manual,* 2nd edn. Geneva: WHO, 2004

World Health Organization. Revised BCG vaccination guidelines for infants at risk for HIV infection. *Wkly Epidem Rec* 2007; 82: 193–6.

Useful addresses

International Union Against Tuberculosis and Lung Disease (The Union)

Department of Tuberculosis Control and Prevention
68 Boulevard Saint-Michel
75006 Paris
France

Website: www.theunion.org
Email: iuatld@theunion.org
Information on tuberculosis can be obtained from: www.tbrieder.org

World Health Organization (WHO)
Stop TB Department (STB)
HIV/AIDS, TB & Malaria Cluster (HTM)
World Health Organization
Avenue Appia 20
1211 Geneva 27
Switzerland

Website: www.who.int/tb/

Information on publications can be found on the website or via email:
publications@who.int

WHO also has many regional offices.

Teaching Aids at Low Cost (TALC)
PO Box 49
St Albans AL1 4AX
UK

TALC is a non-profit organisation set up to promote the health of children and advance medical knowledge and teaching throughout the world by providing and developing educational material for health workers.

Website: www.talcuk.org.
Email: info@talcuk.org

Index

Page numbers in *italics* refer to entries in
tables or figures

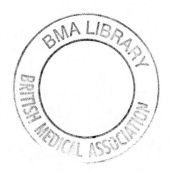